HOW WE SURVIVED
PROSTATE CANCER

HOW WE SURVIVED
PROSTATE CANCER

What We Did and
What We Should Have Done

VICTORIA HALLERMAN

Foreword by Peter S. Albert, M.D.

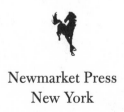

Newmarket Press
New York

This book is published in the United States of America.

FIRST EDITION

ISBN: 978-1-55704-814-1 (hardcover)

10 9 8 7 6 5 4 3 2 1

ISBN: 978-1-55704-819-6 (paperback)

10 9 8 7 6 5 4 3 2 1

Library of Congress Cataloging-in-Publication Data

Hallerman, Victoria.
How we survived prostate cancer : what we did and what we should have done / Victoria Hallerman ; foreword by Peter S. Albert.
p. cm.
Includes bibliographical references and index.
ISBN 978-1-55704-814-1 (hardcover : alk. paper) — ISBN 978-1-55704-819-6 (pbk. : alk. paper) 1. Prostate—Cancer—Popular works. I. Title.
RC280.P7.H35 2009
616.99'463—dc22
2008046354

QUANTITY PURCHASES
Companies, professional groups, clubs, and other organizations may qualify for special terms when ordering quantities of this title. For information or a catalog, write Special Sales Department, Newmarket Press, 18 East 48th Street, New York, NY 10017; call (212) 832-3575; fax (212) 832-3629; or e-mail info@newmarketpress.com.

Designed by Mary Jane Di Massi

Manufactured in the United States of America.

For Alan Rosenthal, gone too soon

CONTENTS

FOREWORD

PROSTATE CANCER is a disease of the aging male. It is rarely seen in men under the age of forty and usually reaches a peak in a man's eighth decade. Uncommon in Asia, Africa, and Latin America, prostate cancer's incidence is highest in the United States and Scandinavia. In fact, it is the second most common male cancer in the U.S. and, with the aging of the American male population, its incidence will continue to rise. The good news is that now, with the advent of PSA screening, we can diagnose the disease in its early stages. If prostate cancer is detected early enough, it is almost always curable.

As a practicing urologist for over thirty years (having treated over 2,500 patients with prostate cancer), I have come to realize that a lack of basic knowledge and general confusion often prevent patients and their families from making logical therapeutic choices. Although it is well known that the prostate is a walnut-shaped gland that lies at the base of the bladder, its sexual role has often been misjudged by men with regard to libido and potency. Effects on urinary function may also come as a surprise to the ill-informed. Realizing how important full education is, the prudent doctor would do well to schedule extra consultation sessions to discuss possible side effects.

How should a patient and his partner or family go about finding the right doctor? A good doctor should also be a good teacher. Such a physician will help the patient and family to understand that healing, as Hippocrates taught, is a matter of time, but also a matter of opportunity. The doctor, the patient, and family or partner will search for and find the right opportunities on their difficult journey through treatment and beyond.

I encourage each patient to go for a second opinion, if possible with a physician who does both surgery and radiation, in the hopes of receiving a fair assessment of the options. Treatment choices should be in partnership and based on the patient's age, medical status, stage of his disease, PSA, and lifestyle. Once the patient, family, and doctor have made their decision, it is wise to go forward and not look back: no second-guessing, no "I wish I had . . . ." This can be damaging to mental health.

Victoria calls her husband's—and her—experience a "cautionary tale." She and Dean *are* looking back, for the purpose of showing others the way. She hopes to steer the newly diagnosed patient and partner clear of some of the pitfalls that she and her husband experienced. She spares nothing in presenting the reader with the hazards of post-diagnosis decision making and the potential side effects during as well as after treatment. By telling her story, she illuminates a plan of attack on prostate cancer that begins with diagnosis and ends in the healing process.

This book is essential for the partner and patient beginning to understand how to survive the treatment of this disease. The concept of a support team for the patient—partner or family and doctor(s) working together—is critical. Victoria, through her own experience, points out the perils of allowing family or partners to be frozen out of consultation. She reminds the reader that if your physician/partner doesn't feel right to you, you may be afraid to ask the right questions. Never hesitate to seek the help of another doctor, or you may end up undergoing a treatment you'll later regret.

It is my hope that in reading this book, the patient and his partner or family faced with many options will find the one treatment that fits the case and be well prepared for a new life beyond treatment.

—Peter S. Albert, M.D.
Staten Island Urological Associates, P.C.
New York

HOW WE SURVIVED
PROSTATE CANCER

All This and Cancer, Too

AFTER THIRTY-NINE years of married life, occupying one half of a king-sized bed, I've made a part-time home for myself in the attic, under the sloped eaves of our house. Most nights my husband sleeps in our bed one flight below. It wasn't ordinary marital discontent or the desire for solitude that drove me up the attic stairs. I didn't go willingly. I miss the rhythms and certainty of sleeping together every night. I miss our big bed, where once we cuddled routinely into sleep; we both miss natural (that is, unpremeditated) sex. We miss those days, and most of all we miss who we were then.

Five years ago, I climbed these attic stairs routinely, but often these days, I find myself sleeping downstairs. Of course it isn't the same: we know we're changed after cancer, after the seeds and the hormone suppressants. In some ways we're stronger, closer, but all those years of habitual nesting, pelvis curved into pelvis, then lights out—that's all gone. Six years since Dean got the news about cancer, a little more than five years since 107 radioactive iodine "seeds" were implanted in his prostate, we're just beginning to find our way back to living, without thinking all the time about cancer or the effects of the cure.

We're the lucky ones, so far still cancer-free. Incontinence has mostly subsided. Dean still takes three drugs: an analgesic for the burning sensation that urination still sometimes causes, a drug to regulate urinary flow, and another to control what he calls his "surges": urinary urges that go nowhere. The scarring that implanted radioactive seeds sometimes cause has implications for erectile function that we never knew about. Not long ago the pain caused by bladder inflammation made him fly out of bed six or eight times in a single night. For at least a year, he seemed like a trout in a skillet full of hot oil. *Sauté*: Isn't that from the French verb "to leap"? He was leaping, all right; his bladder dominated his life for nearly two years. Lying as the gland in question does, at a kind of crossroads in the male body where all the intimate functions meet—urinary, sexual, bowel—the prostate has touchy neighbors. But good news: after about a year and a half, urinary flow became governable again—no more pads to tuck into the briefcase. As long as he remembers to fill those three prescriptions, he's all right, though he still rushes to the restroom after a long car trip.

Libido, spontaneous erectile function? These are still things to reach for, to continue to try to reinvent, six years after it all began.

This book began as a journal to save my wits. It developed into a memoir lamenting the lack of comprehensible information afforded to many patients by modern medicine, and has morphed at last into a cautionary tale regretting the many errors we made as patient and partner. My friend and adviser, Elaine Albert, nurse and trained group facilitator, recently observed, "But you and Dean did everything wrong!" We did. We never got a second or third opinion. We shopped for medicine the way some people shop for expensive shoes—going to the "best" places—and we were disastrously ignorant of treatment aftereffects. This last was a result of bad doctoring, magical thinking, and an unfortunately flawed support group that discouraged any real sense of community. The actual physical result—that biopsies have come and gone and that Dean to date is cancer-free—is our great blessing. But our marriage has only recently begun to crawl out from under the treatment rock that fell on it six years ago. We learned a lot, and every day brings a new lesson. Meanwhile, others can benefit from our training in the school of experience.

New strategies are evolving for treating prostate cancer, but the major treatment choices are still, as they were for us six years ago: prostatectomy (the gland surgically removed); external beam radia-

2

tion (radiation treatments over a course of weeks or months, nowadays taking the form of the more precisely targeted IMRT: intensity modulated radiation therapy); and finally, another form of radiation, the treatment Dean chose, brachytherapy (an outpatient surgical procedure in which radioactive "seeds" are "planted" strategically in the prostate).

Hormone ablation or deprivation—in which the body's production of testosterone is shut down—sometimes assists radiation, serving as a "palliative" treatment. It works this way: since testosterone feeds the growth of prostate cancer cells as gasoline feeds a fire, hormone therapy (reducing testosterone via shots and pills to near zero) is a way of discouraging that growth. It is also used, as in Dean's case, to shrink the prostate in advance of brachytherapy. But this drastic testosterone elimination would, for him, still on the youngish side of fifty-six, prove a particular hell: E.D., mood swings, hot flashes, lethargy, and a total loss of libido.

There is no "best" treatment for prostate cancer (often abbreviated as PCa), no one-size-fits-all. None of the major methods is without hazard for urinary and sexual quality of life, and to make matters more confusing, medical talk on this disease changes daily. For example, there is a sizable contingent of doctors and researchers who now lean in the direction of recommending what is called active surveillance (that is, "watchful waiting")—doing nothing at all, just periodic biopsies—for men whose cancers are at a low stage, as Dean's was. PSA screening itself has come under heavy fire recently. Are we overtreating a large population of men—causing unnecessary incontinence, E.D., and general suffering—when many of these men would live on into old age and die of something else?

Others argue, rightly, that without PSA we don't know which men harbor these cancers, and that approximately 1 man in 10 would probably die of an atypically fast-growing prostate cancer. Some men do choose no treatment at all, after a positive biopsy, but that's hard, too, living with the knowledge of cancer, not knowing if it will accelerate. Dean says that, for all he has been through, he is

(1) glad he knew and (2) without regret at having taken action of some kind. He would never have been happy as a watchful waiter.

That said, knowing what we know now—about prostate size and seed implantation, about the smart way to use the arsenal of medical weapons available to a youngish man—we wish we'd gone for at least a second opinion. Surgical removal of the prostate is often a good treatment choice if the patient is young and healthy enough (sixty-five or under), which reserves radiation for any later recurrence. Ironically, in Dean's case, the hormone treatments undercut any supposed potency-sparing benefits the seeds might have offered.

Dean expects, eventually, to be a treatment "old-timer," like those patients a hundred years ago who received arsenic to combat venereal disease before there was such a thing as penicillin. Wistfully the other day he wondered aloud what it might be like to have a libido again. It isn't just erections that are missing, but the whole idea of sensuality.

We can talk about it now, but not so long ago depression and silence, and a certain resulting distance, chilled our marriage. A woman I recently spoke to confesses to feeling a sadness she wasn't entirely aware of, buried since her husband had his prostatectomy over four years ago. There seemed little time back then to reflect on how their life together had changed. The growing public conversation about quality of life after prostate cancer treatment, however, is changing the way doctors, patients, and partners think about treatment.

But Dean is alive. We celebrate this fact every morning at breakfast, every evening that finds us together in our kitchen or cuddling before lights out, before I either do or don't climb the attic stairs. The writing of this book—together—has been the last and most important aspect of our healing. Dean's voice is an important presence in these pages, the result of many nights he spent alone with an old tape recorder. Most chapters end with the voices of other partners or information about the changing and very public prostate cancer treatment dialogue surrounding treatment and its aftermath, followed by a Practical Guide of tips and information relevant to the chapter. A Glossary at the back of the book defines basic terms.

The attic remains my part-time refuge. What drove me up the chipped green stairs initially was Dean's need to be alone. Then my makeshift apartment became the one place where I could be an individual, not half of a perilously balanced duo. Every Wednesday night I could complain to my therapist. I also had my TV, my claw-foot bathtub, a radio, a work desk for my computer, my teapot, and a jar of biscotti. One flight below, Dean had his own room, the solitude he needed to work things out, and the telephone network of men he talked to every night who were up late undergoing similar ordeals. That's how he wanted it; some men do.

In many ways we're closer than ever: the conversation, the doorway kiss, the cuddle that curves us into sleep on those nights we spend together. Then he touches my nose in the dark, in hopes that I'll stop snoring, and I remember my room, and I want a bath and my book, after all.

My attic retreat, these days, feels very much like the third floor of my parents' house, which I had to myself as a shy teenager. In that sense, my fondness for it may be a regression—perhaps, as an old friend, a clinical psychologist, used to say, "regression in the service of the ego." The ego needs rest and solitude—and perspective. So here I am, sleeping occasionally through the night downstairs, but often, as late as dawn, getting up and climbing the stairs to settle into my own bed and watch the sun drag its orange light once more over the Brooklyn shore.

Who are we now? That's the question I'm chewing on these days. Beyond that, and back there somewhere, *Who were we?* Born in Cincinnati, we met, married, and ran off to the East Coast, both barely of legal age. We settled in Staten Island, ultimately in this house, on a hill overlooking New York Harbor. We've lived here for better than thirty years. He's sixty-two now, and I am sixty. My birthday is in February, his is in May—so for a brief time every year, we seem to be closer in age; then I'm tailing him again, as he gains another year. We've been married thirty-nine years. He's a business-man and I'm a poet, a teacher. That's a glimpse, but certain signifi-cant details are missing; without them, it would be hard to say why we're still in love, and why cancer—with all of its bluster and treat-ment complications—hasn't after all divided us.

Aside from cancer, the other physical thing you need to know about my husband is that he lives in a world somewhere between blindness and sight. He has been in this peculiar realm since I've known him, although he spent the first fifteen and a half years nor-mally sighted. Call him what you may: legally blind, visually impaired, partially sighted, visually handicapped, even disabled. He's okay with any of these terms, though he prefers "handi-capped"—it appeals to the sporting nature in him—and he loathes "differently abled." "It's different, all right," he says.

Struck at the age of fifteen with sudden macular degeneration (Stargardt's disease), he copes with a little under 4 percent normal vision to this day. In Cincinnati, where we were both born and raised, doctors failed to properly diagnose his condition. Among other factors, the technology simply wasn't in place. His parents went from doctor to doctor looking for a solution. Dean often felt like an oddity, a specimen. The doctors having failed to diagnose a rare genetic condition, Dean's parents sent him to a psychotherapist for several anguished years. When he was grown, he promised him-self, he wouldn't rely on anyone—friend or family member—for help in taking care of his own health. He has kept that promise until recently, until cancer. He thought he could handle prostate cancer on his own, but nobody should make a cancer treatment decision alone.

I met Dean a little more than two years after his vision "went." Eighteen and idealistic, I found his courage and his inventiveness—which still causes thoughtless strangers to blurt, "But you don't look blind!"—amazing, a reason to fall in love. His resilience and determination to make it in a sighted world, and on his own, continue to astonish and move me. The fact of his near-blindness has colored his, and our, whole life.

We married and moved from Cincinnati to New York City when I was barely twenty-one. We were both running away from parents, a running that became a distance race and has had something to do with the longevity of our relationship. The year was 1969; we were married as feminism hit its stride. I took back my single name six months after we moved to New York, transfixed by *The Second Sex*. For a time, early on, we took off our rings: we both wanted so badly to be thought of as individuals! And individuals we have remained; the space we each seem to need within marriage is a good thing, but delicate in the balancing.

So many lives within one long life together: we have each tried on a variety of costumes in the thirty-nine years since we drove away from Cincinnati. In the process of becoming a poet and writer, I have worked as an afterschool art instructor for young children, a chef's assistant, a bookkeeper, a theater manager, and even, in my earliest years, a dog walker. In my forties, I became an educator, using poetry to further literacy, working as a teacher and literacy staff developer in New York's public schools.

Radio, Dean had imagined, might be a good career choice for a man who could go blind at any moment. Before we left Cincinnati he completed his degree in Radio/Television. It was film, then video and Web sites—corporate communications—he finally settled on, falling back, remarkably, on the visual aspects of his education. He began at a "youth marketing firm" in New York, then went to work in the early 70s at Joko Films (John Lennon and Yoko Ono's creative film venture). At his next job he produced telethons for Geraldo Rivera's hip 70s charity, One to One, founded to get children out of Willowbrook, the infamous state institution. After several other show business ventures, he ran two large corporate television departments, then founded his own business communications firm.

There were no children. With art and business and a major handicap, our life together was already complicated enough.

We've started over so many times, and in each instance it has been the brilliant salesman, the entrepreneur, the producer, the man who may go blind any minute, who should have gone blind entirely at sixteen, who continues to astonish his doctors, that man who pulls, at the last minute, $2,000 in hundred-dollar bills one at a time out of his pants pockets, or hands over the folded, wrinkled check for twenty grand.

He has been known to edit video and film, with his precious 4 percent vision, and to call the camera shots for live shows—nobody knows quite how. As for me, despite (these days) severe osteoarthritis, I still get around our three-story house, fetch and carry groceries and dry cleaning, all the stuff I've always done, just more slowly and with some considerable pain. I rub away his vision headaches, he massages my aching shoulder, legs, and back. What would we do without each other? We struggle to contain it all, our life—who we were, who we are: all this and cancer, too.

CHAPTER ONE

CROSSING THE CANCER DIVIDE:
Words You Hoped You'd Never Hear

> About suffering they were never wrong,
> The Old Masters: how well they understood
> Its human position; how it takes place
> While someone else is eating or opening a window
> or just walking dully along.
>
> —from "Musée des Beaux Arts," W. H. Auden

SEPTEMBER 2002 WAS the last innocent month of our lives. At least it started out that way; I think of it as "the month of not-knowing," mauve with a tinge of rust, colors of the mountains where I'd traveled on a trip west with a group of old friends, fellow poets. Mauve and rust are the eternal colors of those mountains; they signal the year's turning. *Fall* is such a ripe and dangerous word. The leaves are falling, of course, so are the temperature and the daylight— falling to dusk closer to six than to seven.

Progress toward the bleak season seemed well under way those ten days I spent in Montana. September is like October in New York, a foretaste for the eastern traveler. We were glad of our scarves, gloves, and socks, astonished to see our breath so soon. I was traveling with six women, close friends, who meet every other week from fall through spring, a writing workshop group that evolved from our study with the same poet twenty-nine years ago. We've been meeting for exactly that long, going on retreat together, usually to a local beach house. But 2002 was different: the first anniversary of the 9/11 attacks. One of our oldest members, who had watched from her apartment window as the towers fell, had left, suddenly—in large part to achieve emotional distance from the disaster—settling in Missoula, Montana.

To honor her we planned a train adventure, but while the others flew there, saving the train for the journey home, I wanted the whole experience. So I went by myself as far as Chicago on "The Empire Builder." After a brief visit with my niece in Evanston, I flew the last leg to Missoula. I was the first to arrive. The airport was tiny, and charmingly bizarre: luggage carousels topped with stuffed grizzlies and huge mountain lions, their still eyes staring out from glass cases, posed in attitudes of attack, each a life removed.

One by one, the others arrived, and we settled in to our week together, exploring the area between Whitefish and Missoula, meeting daily to discuss our poems, going out for food at night, then back to our rooms to write.

In Glacier National Park, we talked about heaven as we clung to the curves of a road called Going-to-the-Sun. A river at the base of the canyon seemed small as a trickle at the bottom of a deep tub. My ears popped now and then from the altitude. We looked for moose and bear, but never saw another living creature. It was the last day the park was open, with great, sad fires—the last of the season—in the lodges we stopped at.

IN DEAN'S WORDS

In the summer of 2001, my PSA had begun to rise; I'd had to be told what a PSA was—checked, the doctor noted, routinely over the past several years. Toward the end of that summer, my primary care physician had recommended a urologist who, because of his prominence in a particular hospital, was a conduit to "one of the best radiation oncologists in New York," just in case. I didn't tell Vicki—no cause for alarm yet. I went to the urologist, the first one I'd ever visited. We monitored my PSA as it climbed—and climbed.

In September 2001, I had my first biopsy. I told Vicki we were just being careful, and, no, it wasn't necessary for her to come along to the doctor with me. There never seemed to be any other wives or partners in the waiting room there, and I felt competent to do these things on my own. The biopsy was terrifying to me, and it hurt: he took six or more core samples, through the anus, each clipped by a special device. The sensation of each "clip" is what I imagine it feels like to be kicked in the stomach by a horse; I bled a lot afterward.

Six days later the results came back negative. *Whew.* I can still tell you the exact phone booth in the Cincinnati airport I was standing at when the doctor's receptionist said, "Oh, everything's just fine."

Ignorant of what Dean was going through back home, I sat on the edge of Going-to-the-Sun Road and took in the glacial landscape, my idea of the hereafter. In all the group, I was the only one, it seemed, who thought of heaven as a solitude. But how quickly solitude can flip into the hell of isolation, something I would come to know all too well in the months that followed.

It was a delicious adventure all the way home from Whitefish, Montana, to New York City by train, this time in the company of my friends. Dean, on my cell phone over the great distance, sang me funny little songs that crackled in the earpiece as "The Lake Shore Limited" slugged east to Chicago; there we boarded my old friend, "The Empire Builder," and Dean tracked our progress, met us at the station with a redcap, helped us sort our baggage. He was, as always, generous and welcoming.

At dinner the night of my return, we talked of everything but. He did not tell me his news. Not until six days later, halfway through some ears of corn, did he finally blurt it. He hardly let a breath pass between "I have prostate cancer" and "but it's almost 100 percent

IN DEAN'S WORDS

Through all this, I'd been "brave" and kept my misery from Vicki. Who wants to talk about his anus? Then, my PSA went from 6.8 to 7.3 to 8.1 to 8.7 to 9.2 to 10.1 and then 10.6. "Another biopsy?"

"It's the only way," the doctor explained.

"There's gotta be a less painful procedure," I pleaded.

It turned out that he'd known about a pain-killing refinement for some time. I should have gotten the message then; compassion was not this man's strong suit. But he was the conduit to the famous radiation oncologist, so I stayed in there. This time, he used a special Novocaine needle device before the procedure, so the second biopsy was a nearly painless experience. Vicki left for Montana a few days afterward. I hadn't even told her I was having another one; why worry her? Four days later, I got the bad news.

curable." He wanted to defang the beast right in front of me, let me know he knew how to handle things.

I dropped my fork, and the room tilted a little. It felt like an earth tremor I once lived through in a restaurant in Mexico City, when, just for a moment, the chandeliers tilted. I don't remember what I said, but I do remember looking down into the conversation, as from a great height. I was scared. Later, I would feel betrayed; why hadn't he trusted me to help?

Always the first to have an opinion on any subject, I was shocked this time into near silence. I'd loved this man for so many years, walked the edge of blindness with him, nursed him through a near-fatal appendectomy ten years earlier, and now cancer. Why had he kept all this from me? He said he had the whole thing under control, but I was scared. What exactly is a *prostate*, anyhow? How many wives would know? I didn't voice my anger; I did say, "Oh, Dean," or something to that effect. I came over and sat next to him, but already something had divided us.

He had cancer. Only minutes before, we had been—or so it seemed—two reasonably healthy people, and now we were looking at each other across a divide. After a long while, I think I said, "What can I do?" Then, "Why didn't you tell me?" He already had a treatment lined up, he said, seeds and hormone therapy, and he believed this combined strategy to be the best course. I was back to square one, absorbing the fact that he'd had a second biopsy.

Here we were, husband and wife, the afflicted and the unafflicted, the one threatened, the other apparently spared. To borrow from Susan Sontag's *Illness as Metaphor*, Dean had begun his journey out from the shore of good health; I stood, watching his sudden departure.

Brachytherapy, he assured me, was the best choice—the implantation of radioactive seeds in the gland itself—combined with hormone ablation to reduce testosterone levels to near zero. Testosterone, he explained, makes it easier for prostate cancer to grow.

IN DEAN'S WORDS

It was so easy not to tell. In fact, if I didn't say anything, then it wasn't real. I meant to tell her a hundred or more times—at dinner, across breakfast, in a telephone call—no, you can't tell her over the phone. Dinner the night after? No, friends are showing up. Finally one night, about six days after, it tumbled out of me over dinner, just the two of us, candlelight. I couldn't see her across the table, but somehow I felt her go ashen. Her mouth, I think, fell open, and her eyes—what I could see of them—seemed to darken. She hesitated for only a moment. I filled that moment: "But I know exactly what I'm going to do."

WHAT WE KNOW NOW

Fresh from diagnosis, what Dean didn't fully understand was that if you use radiation first, it is almost impossible to do surgery second, should there be a recurrence. Apparently nobody had told him this—but then, he'd gone alone to appointments and perhaps didn't remember everything or ask the right questions. As for hormone treatments, his urologist hadn't fully explained, or Dean hadn't fully understood, the significance of his oversized prostate (90.3 grams). In such cases, hormone treatments do more than simply discourage cancer. By causing the gland to shrink to a viable size, they make implantation possible for men with large prostates.

So the decision had been made, and who could argue? I could have. Should have. I wanted to help him research the cures, visit his urologist, but he seemed to have it all sewn up. Among Dean's greatest talents is his ability to argue persuasively; he is, among other things in his professional life, a crack salesman. And so, he sold me on the idea of this treatment, the hot new cure, endorsed by famous men still active in public life (Giuliani, the embattled mayor; a few prominent football players): the seeds. Seeds mean life, and those in charge of marketing brachytherapy know the attractiveness of the metaphor: he'd bought it, this cure, then sold it to me. Behind his sales pitch was his lifelong need to handle his own health issues.

As to the prostate gland, what did I know? If asked, I'm sure I would have said that it has something to do with a man's sperm. Actually, as I subsequently learned, the prostate is one of the male body's main sources of hormone; it adds vital nutrients and fluid to the sperm, making it possible to father children. (For details about the prostate's role, see chapter 12 and the Glossary.) Way back in high school, divided according to sex, we girls had looked at one set of cutaways—the uterus, the fallopian tubes—while, presumably, the boys in the room across the hall were looking at penises, scrotums, and perhaps this mysterious gland. That peculiar form of segregation in high school was preparing me for marriage the good old-fashioned way: the girls and the boys, a subtle division, one I'm sure other female partners of prostate sufferers have contended with. We all have hearts, lungs, brains, and stomachs; when those organs are threatened in a partner of the opposite sex, we're equipped, literally, to understand. I suppose men who hear that their wives have ovarian or uterine cancer must go through a similar confusion. What's it like to be a man? A woman? One of the things that draws men and women together as lovers is physical difference. Just how important is testosterone in a man's daily life? We were about to find out.

IN DEAN'S WORDS

First thing one morning, Erin at work urged, "Call your urologist right away—he's been calling pretty insistently." Then the doctor's receptionist seemed to have no time for the usual pleasantries, just put me right through.

This urologist, never affable, seemed suddenly nervous and chatty, determined to slow things down with small talk, but I rushed the question.

"You have some bad news for me?"

"Well now, not so terrible, but your biopsy did come back positive."

Positive/negative—do the reversal thing: positive *means bad.*

"You can come in at your convenience sometime next week; no need to rush."

"There is, too! I have cancer!"

I made an appointment for the next morning. Then I put the phone down and just stood there. I had made the call in

15

my office with the door closed, standing up the whole time. I'd been visible through the glass partition all along. Erin knocked at my door, violating an office rule that protects privacy, then opened it and crossed halfway to the desk.

"Are you all right?"

"No. No, I'm not all right."

I was leaning on the desk for support.

"You were standing there twenty-three minutes," she observed.

It had seemed like four minutes, maybe five, and for a few of those minutes the sofa on the other side of the room had seemed to be sliding; the room had turned slightly, counter-clockwise.

I left the table that night feeling scared and confused, missing Dean, as if he'd suddenly gone far away. While I had been tooling through Glacier Park or looking placidly out the windows of a train, he'd been on a private journey through hell. It had been a misplaced, if compelling, survival strategy on his part not to tell me. If I didn't know, then he could pretend he'd never heard. I had been behind the one-way glass, and he could see in. My innocence had been his escape.

Now there was no escape for either of us. He decided not to go for treatments right away; he had "everything under control." Fall was just starting, business picking up, and we had already made our Key West reservations for December, our yearly vacation. He wanted everything to remain the same. The egg of denial has a thin, strong shell: it simply hadn't cracked yet. Somehow, he knew enough to know that hormone therapy would change things. Hot flashes, depression, erectile dysfunction, lethargy, possible weight gain, breast swelling: the urologist had mentioned these. But, optimist that Dean tends to be, he had convinced himself—and me—

IN DEAN'S WORDS

I don't recall what I did that night—watch baseball, cuddle the dogs. Don't know whether my insomnia is worse these days, as a result of cancer, but that weekend I remember waking up often in the middle of the night, thinking, "I can't sleep and I have cancer," then thinking, "Last week at this time, I would've just said, 'I can't sleep.'"

Ever play that game when you were a kid, adding the same phrase to everything you say? We ate dinner . . . under the blanket. We played together . . . under the blanket. Made everything a raunchy eighth-grade joke. Well, that happened to me after I got the news. "I'm going to work now . . . and I have cancer." "This chocolate is delicious . . . and I have cancer."

Vicki called that night and the other nights, but how could I tell her? She didn't have that phrase attaching itself to everything she said or thought. She was free, for a while. There was something else, too. I took the time to learn to live with this thing. I was scared, yes, but not terrified. I knew I had a pretty good chance with this thing—slow moving as it often is—of surviving into some kind of old age, but cancer's an awful kind of knowledge, and I'd been living on the edge of it for a long time, going for biopsies, my PSA rising all along. By the time her train rolled into Penn Station that night eight days later, I was ready to tell her, would've told her if we'd been alone, but all the others were there: chatting, hugging, taking pictures, looking for pieces of luggage. So then, I thought I'd tell her in the cab on the way home, but it wasn't private enough, and then at home . . . well, there is no good time for bad news. I just kept putting it off.

that these effects would be temporary. As for libido, either the doctor hadn't mentioned it or Dean had failed to hear, a classic example of why cancer patients should never enter the doctor's office alone.

Key West would be the journey before the journey. Before flying to Florida, we were scheduled to meet with the revered radiation oncologist who would assemble the team that would "plant" the seeds. We had granted ourselves a little time to wait and absorb—a good thing for quality of life as it turned out, though not without hazard. While waiting, we both now wish we had done some research.

I browsed the shelves of various bookstores, in that passive, reticent state I'd fallen into, the complement to his "I know what I'm doing." These days, I would have Googled everything but, always technologically retrograde, I was downright naive back then, so I wandered in bookstores from Health to Self-Help looking for something, anything. I found either falsely cheerful texts about procedures or charts and graphs and lots of confusing medical language.

The seeds are no fraud: they have a respectable track record, but the other two main treatment strategies, equally recommended by prominent doctors, should have been the second and third opinions Dean never got. A rival institution in our area promotes prostatectomy—the "nerve-sparing" removal of the prostate. External beam radiation (or these days, IMRT: intensity modulated radiation therapy) requires steady visits to a radiologist, but would not have required the shrinking of Dean's large prostate. But neither rival treatment would have allowed him to continue his work life unabated, with its constant travel schedule and the demands of running a small communications company. As I revisit those last days of September, I think that's probably why he clung to brachytherapy so steadfastly.

All that fall was an unwitting goodbye, for both of us, to a lot of things: to the assumption each night that we would sleep together, to unpremeditated sex, to natural erectile function, to medically

IN DEAN'S WORDS

I was sitting on a park bench across from the hospital after the bone and CT scans watching all these children playing with their nannies and parents. There was that clear gold autumn light, almost like Paris. They'd packed me full of barium, seemed like gallons of it. I was feeling pretty lonely, and very sorry for myself. I wish I'd known how bad it could be—worse than a biopsy, the scans to find out where else cancer might be hiding in my body.

unaided continence. He knew this therapy would change him, and I knew it would change us, though neither of us understood quite how. Despite what the doctors were saying, we sensed treatment would be neither quick nor efficient. How can the placement of radioactive pellets in flesh be a simple thing? How can the virtual elimination of something as vital as testosterone fail to affect quality of life? Side effects, in our case, would prove to have been greatly underestimated.

Meanwhile, it was as if he had gotten up and moved into the room next door. His lifelong need to overcome his own health problems, my ignorance and passivity, the urologist's lack of compassion and poor communication skills, and our joint sense of denial combined to create a volatile setting for our crisis and to increase the sense of isolation and helplessness we each felt. I knew he was over there; I could hear and see him through the partition that separated us: the cancer, and his proposed cure, "the protocols." This language of medicine was another divider. Dean was moving away from life as we had known it.

Joint discussions with the doctor—which I failed to request, Dean seemed unable to suggest, and his urologist never offered— would perhaps have narrowed the growing gap between us. Susan Sontag observes this separation as a natural progress of disease:

19

those who have been seriously ill have dual citizenship in both lands, the land of illness and the land of health. Some people are permanent expatriates, living forever in the space created by their illness, while others cross back over into health. But their experience, their travels, so to speak, give them another dimension. The language of science—*positive, negative, biopsy, core sample, PSA, Gleason*—and the marks chronic pain leaves on the psyche, combined with certain physical limitations imposed by treatment, have changed them forever.

As I was moving through the Montana mountains, so cold and mysteriously lacking in animal life, he was entering his own new landscape. Returning, I joined him there, as close as I could get. *If only I had stayed home.* He would have come up the steps, the awful night of the day he got his news, and I would have been there. He would have told me right off. Then September would have been "the month of knowing" for both of us, perhaps even "the month of second opinions."

How can I forgive myself for pleasure while my lover was in agony? But you must, ultimately. Beyond that, how can I forgive my lover for not sharing his misery with me more completely? You must do that too, and sooner.

Mauve and rust are the colors that gave me this remembrance of a particular September. They belong to Glacier, to the mountains we drove through, but they also belong to what I didn't know. In my personal prism, mauve seems a color not to be trusted, one that changes with the light, a purple so pale it could turn gray or pink, deceptive, like stories withheld, treatments attractively packaged. And rust? Well, that's the color of biopsy, of needle tests, and death, the final divider.

Many of the poems I have written since that September have divisions in them: walls, sealed boxes, isolated rooms, cells. Cancer did this to us. It isn't a contagion, but the idea of it is infectious. It can change the way you think about yourself, about your lover, the

20

way your lover thinks about you. If you're the patient, your death or the possibility of it becomes your new companion; cancer can appear at any time. If you're the partner of someone who's been diagnosed, the treatment experience reminds you absolutely that we die. Beyond that experience is a healing time, a time for getting back to daily living. But that September, we were voyaging out, and couldn't imagine the return trip.

A CONVERSATION WITH EVE

When I began this book, I was convinced I was telling "the wife's story" or, as one friend put it, "prostate cancer from the distaff side." There is, I have discovered, no such universal story. About two years ago I sat in on a meeting of Side by Side, a women's prostate cancer support group (affiliated with a chapter of Man to Man). After the meeting I wrote in my notebook, "This process is mostly about loss and survival." The next day I interviewed Eve, a stylish woman in her early sixties. She had met Harry at an art gallery and they'd flirted. Their second date was on the day he got his news.

"We've just celebrated six years together," she bragged happily over tea in a local coffeehouse. "We sort of dated around the local art scene: we were both fanatics for painting—the New York school, mostly. I'd had my eye on him, thought he was really cute. So we went to a show, and then he asked me if I wanted to come back to his place. We had a drink or two and talked. The next night we had dinner at his apartment—he's a great cook—and he said, 'You know, before this goes any further, I think there's something you ought to know . . . . I've just had a positive biopsy—it's prostate cancer. So if you want to get up right now and walk out the door. . . . '"

She considered it. "For me it was a dilemma; I was thinking, 'Well, yes, I could, couldn't I? I could just walk out and pretend this didn't happen.' But then what I said to him was, 'Let me be your friend through this; let me be one of the people you can count on.' I didn't know what to expect; I hadn't been through this with anybody else."

Harry did extensive research; he got two or three differing opinions and read up on all the possible treatments; he attended a few meetings of a local discussion group, then he booked a trip to consult a well-known oncologist hours away, somebody who knew about all the options but didn't have, in his words, "any kind of bias." A radical prostatectomy was his choice, and Eve fell happily into her supporting role, the more-than-casual friend. I asked her if she'd followed the details of his treatment. "Not really . . . I just read the things that he gave me to read and familiarized myself with the choices, especially the one he had made. It's kind of funny to me now. Cancer and our relationship started at the same time. So we didn't have a 'before' to compare this 'after' to."

Why did this idea seem so familiar to me? Wasn't she like the girl I'd been, nearly forty years ago, falling in love with a man who had just gone nearly blind? The sparkles in his retina had been, and continue to be, part of us. I have never known the Dean of sixteen and before, the man with 20/20 vision. After talking to Eve I took out my notebook and crossed out the sentence about loss and survival, the one thing I had been convinced we partners of prostate cancer sufferers all have in common. In its place I scribbled—in admiration, tinged with a bit of envy—"Eve has lost nothing."

CHAPTER TWO

A RUSH OF INFORMATION:

First Month Alone Together with Cancer

OCTOBER

Now that we knew Dean had cancer, we didn't tell a soul. The idea had occurred to us separately but simultaneously. We gave cancer a nickname, "Hitler." We would beat him, push him back, without family or friends even knowing there'd been a war on.

We went about our lives as usual, making winter vacation plans, holing ourselves up in our cabin near the shore those weekends, the light austere as it always is in October, forbiddingly clear that year.

Against the urgings of his urologist, Dean postponed treatment protocols until January, after our annual vacation in Key West. He needed, he said, some time to reflect, prepare. Somehow we must have known how profoundly our lives would change during and after treatment, but we couldn't talk about it.

Falsely brave we were, lost in October's darkening forest. Yellow, crimson, russet, bronze, and brown—colors of the tree-lined Merritt Parkway, colors I have always loved, but that October dreaded: the slow descent into winter, the blank white season, and whatever lay beyond. Back and forth we went on the Merritt to Connecticut, using up those few warm weekends and, though we didn't know it, the last of our healthy, carefree middle years.

We were fifty-somethings who looked and felt forty. Passive in response to a distant and well-connected doctor who seemed to be telling us everything would be fine after a certain amount of unpleasantness, we just went along. One month in, what should we have been doing? Research, for one thing. Building a support network, for another.

Waterlight reflected off the Sound, on the pine ceiling above our bed, on Saturday mornings, while the dogs stirred and rolled over on the floor nearby. Dean recalls the weekends that month seeming "to glide by, going way too fast: football, first fires in the hearth, long, dusty walks through ankle-deep leaves," to be followed by winter . . . and what we couldn't yet acknowledge: the slow winnowing of testosterone with its subtle and not-so-subtle changes, then in spring the seeds, radiation that would leave scars of all kinds.

We were scared, deliberately ignorant, but the dogs knew something was up. We had a sixteen-year-old Lab (Cheeno, short for Cappuccino) and a greyhound–pit bull mix (Audrey), about seven years old. After trundling north to the Connecticut shore once a week in the station wagon, the four of us started each day sitting on the porch, then ended it with fish, grilled on the fire. Lame, Cheeno could barely stagger around the yard.

Back in the city, Dean discouraged me from coming with him on several urology appointments, a decision he now regrets. The one

IN DEAN'S WORDS

Cheeno was an old dog. I think he grew very wise that fall, if a dog could be said to be wise. It seemed to me that when he looked at me, he knew we were both in for a struggle. At the same time, I remember thinking, "You just can't die on me—not this year." What clearer reminder of your own death can you have than this animal who'd been at the center of your life for fifteen years, now barely able to stand up?

time I did come, I felt entirely unwelcome, like an intruder. But for the receptionist, I never saw another woman in that office.

Brachytherapy was all the rage that year, made famous by New York's Mayor Rudy Giuliani and his radiation oncologist, planter of celebrity "seeds."

An ad in *The New Yorker* boasted:

Prostate Surgery	[seed] Treatment
• Months of recovery	• Approximately 45-minute procedure
• Higher risk of incontinence	• Recovery in about 2–3 days
• Higher risk of impotence	• One happy significant other

. . . ***Remember*** [product name]. ***Forget the cancer.***

Forget the cancer? Nobody does that, ever. And that "happy significant other"? Even then I felt trivialized. Also, this ad encourages wrong thinking in patients: that sex is performance, that a partner is happy only if that performance is perfectly youthful, just as before.

WHAT WE KNOW NOW

Going alone to appointments, at least the initial ones, is a big mistake. You hear things differently when you've been told your body harbors a cancer, and the myriad treatments, not to mention their technical aspects, are confusing. Some men apparently bring whole family groups for post-biopsy consultations—the more listeners the better! Some couples bring tape recorders, to catch what both might miss. I know now, from monthly support group meetings, that men who go alone on their initial appointments often seem not to know the most rudimentary aspects of their own treatment protocols.

I had, I felt, no power to intervene, no knowledge—or confidence. Since the day he'd told me his news, as I bit down on that last innocent ear of September corn, my silence had become an enchantment. He had already made up his mind, and who was I to object? Who was I? Half of two people whose lives were about to change. Abandon silence, I tell the old me, the one locked in this story. Say everything that is on your mind. If you are terrified, if you are confused, tell him. He's terrified, too.

We'd heard stories of competing treatments that hadn't gone as well as the patient had hoped. A friend had had a prostatectomy several years before and had lost erectile function as well as continence. Besides, Dean urged one Saturday driving north, that operation took a long time for healing, and would be career-altering for a sole proprietor of a small business in difficult fiscal times. As for beam radiation—the third major treatment protocol then—business travel would, Dean thought, frustrate daily treatments.

He was nowhere near ready to quit, more driven than most fully sighted men or women in similar circumstances. I told myself over and over the tale of his life: driven to prove himself in a sighted world, ambitious and determined to make enough money to last the final thirty years of our lives. The seeds seemed so much less intrusive, with their advertised promise of continence, potency, and a quick return to daily routine.

Hormone therapy—the preliminary treatment, to begin in January, after Key West—seemed, in the clear but refracted light of our denial, like a temporary inconvenience: a few hot flashes, some depression. Urged to watch his weight (lethargy and weight gain are possible side effects), Dean gave me the sense, from his consultations with the doctor, that hormone ablation would be nothing more than an unpleasant interval.

In fact, it would prove to be the greatest single life change, beyond macular degeneration, that Dean had ever experienced, one we failed to understand and were emotionally unprepared for. *What were we thinking—or not thinking?* Hot flashes, lethargy, and passivity in a man still active in the push and pull of New York business—we were just hoping it would all be over soon. And nobody mentioned libido. Well, the doctor should have, but we should have asked for details, names of people to talk to. We didn't want to know.

He'd be fine. I told myself that daily, then I told him. Still, I did a few quiet researches on my own. They left me baffled, more confused than ever. The serious texts were extremely clinical, with statistics that seemed impossible to interpret; the anecdotal material wasn't clinical enough. No treatment seemed to guarantee leaving erectile and urinary functions untouched.

Meeting a friend to see a Broadway play, I spent some time book shopping, looking for the guide I'd heard about on prostate cancer written partly for the wives of newly diagnosed patients. At the bookstore a young woman sent me on my way: "Oh, you're on the wrong floor—that would be in Health, the cancer shelf, down on two. Take the escalator." So cancer has a shelf! I mused, the sliding stairs disappearing under my feet one at a time. I found the book, among other titles: *Prostate Cancer for Dummies; The ABC's of Prostate Cancer; The Prostate, a Guide for Men and the Women Who Love Them,* by Dr. Patrick Walsh . . . that was the one.

WHAT WE KNOW NOW

There is no "best" treatment for prostate cancer, no single text or Web site adequate to prepare a man or his partner for the cacophony of recommended treatment regimens and their aftereffects. There is no method, including the seeds, that guarantees anything resembling "normal" life after treatment. There are, however, more and more groups these days and there are ListServs and close-knit online communities. In these contexts, you still might not hear what you need to hear, but nobody should be as alone as we were, or as ignorant.

I took myself out to a tiny elegant bar on Forty-sixth Street, a tall glass of white burgundy for company. I had my own small black easy chair and a place near the window, open to the street, the kind of situation I usually enjoy with a far different kind of book.

Like certain high school texts from long ago, this hefty volume offered lots of technical illustrations, but instead of uteruses and breasts, there were line drawings of penises and cutaways of the prostate. Despite the title, ". . . and the Women Who Love Them," I found little comfort in its pages. We women who love "them" were, it seemed, expected to get out our spiral notebooks and prepare for a pop quiz. I did have my notebook in hand. But where in this book was the advice for me on how to cope with what seemed likely to change our lives forever? Women routinely read about health—theirs and their partners'—and the book was targeting me, but only as a caregiver: how to read up, for him. But I needed something, too. Where were the stories of other women who had gone this way before?

Suddenly, the illustrations seemed like caricatures, like cartoons of rectal exams. It was no good skimming this kind of book in a bar. It didn't help that the author, a famous doctor, is not a proponent of the seed method at all. There is no guaranteed cure, he asserts. True! But I didn't want to hear this.

"We have the best treatment, don't we?" a frightened inner voice intruded. Dr. Walsh would beg to differ. So it's Dr. Walsh for prostatectomy, Dean's urologist for seed implantation, and somebody else—who? I wondered—for beam radiation. Walsh seemed to think the removal of the prostate the only reliable method of avoiding cancer recurrence. And there are, he warns, no re-do's: if cancer returns, prostatectomy isn't a reliable option for former seed patients.

This is what I learned from that book: that I/we knew even less about the prostate, about Gleason grades and statistical likelihoods, than I had feared; that there is no "best" cure—perhaps no cure at all, not exactly.

Dean was stage T1c (PSA 12.8, Gleason 6—see Glossary for definitions). Dr. Walsh seemed to be saying that, for this stage, Dean's planned treatment wasn't the best choice: "Doctors have become highly sophisticated in targeting and placing these radioactive seeds. But do they work? The bottom line is: Not as well as radical prostatectomy or external-beam radiation therapy."

The statistics are tricky to interpret, and each treatment selection process depends on the man, his age, the size of his prostate, his Gleason grade and PSA, his physical robustness, and, to a lesser degree, personal characteristics, such as susceptibility to burning and scarring. There is still no one best way, although Dean's age, relative vigor, large prostate size, and mid-range Gleason grade might have indicated prostatectomy.

Sitting in that long-ago lounge with a tall-stemmed glass that October, I was completely beyond my depths. I felt dizzy; the page blurred for a moment. I closed the book and paid for the glass of wine, late for *A Long Day's Journey into Night*.

My journey, our journey, getting ready for winter, not just any winter. "Go along and it will be over soon," my controlling inner voice whispered. I tried to believe. Not telling anybody still seemed the only power we had over cancer.

WHAT WE KNOW NOW

We could have been sharing our news with the men and women in monthly support group meetings at the hospital. I wish we had had those second Mondays of every month to steady us back then. Emotional isolation is devastating; it magnifies the confusion and the terror that follow diagnosis.

October ends in what was once a beginning, the Celtic New Year, Halloween, El Dia de los Muertos in Mexico. In Aztec and Celtic cultures, the last day in October is when the ghosts of that

WHAT WE KNOW NOW

In his book *Second Opinions*, Jerome Groopman observes, "There are dark corners to every clinical situation. Knowledge in medicine is imperfect. No diagnostic test is flawless. No drug is without side effects, expected or idiosyncratic. No prognosis is fully predictable." Would any other treatment have left Dean with a greater sense of wholeness? Perhaps not. But not rushing to judgment, going for second or third opinons, we would have known we'd had a choice. And finding a doctor we could get along with—that would have changed everything.

year take their final walk. For the living, it's a turning into the new. I have always loved this primitive dark holiday with its carved faces and candles, its sweets to mollify tricksters.

Because Dean and I are childless, each Halloween he spends a lot of money on giant-sized bars of chocolate he gives away with abandon. So our house is known in the neighborhood, and, despite the twenty-five steps to our porch from the street, all manner of jesters, ghosts, and mermaids make their pilgrimage to get a giant Snickers or Milky Way.

That October 31st was no different from others at the end of the evening: chocolate supplies greatly diminished, the candle in the terra-cotta pumpkin burned to a stub. But the night air seemed to be tinged that evening with a sharper than usual flavor. As Dean recalls, "Something of youth was dying."

Can you pause in your cancer treatments to grieve the loss of innocent, almost perfect health? Yes you can, and we should have.

The previous weekend, we'd closed the cabin in Connecticut for the summer and settled in at home with the dogs. I'd decided by then that I couldn't live without telling someone, so I chose one friend, not my oldest and closest, but someone I felt I could trust. Dean was angry, but he came around in time.

I knew this friend was the right one to confide in. Not only is she a good listener and sympathetic, but I wanted the name of her psychotherapist. I knew I couldn't get through the crisis without professional help. It was exploding in me, this news; the phone line was the end of a long fuse.

"Dean has prostate cancer," I fired off to her, breaking the silence.

"What is uttered," according to Thomas Mann, "is finished and done with." Or, in this case, begun.

THE LATEST SCOOP ON PSA

What exactly is PSA, the main screening tool for prostate cancer in the United States? Levels of *prostate-specific antigen,* a glyco-protein normally released by prostate cells into the bloodstream, rise in the blood early in the course of a cancer. That seems simple enough, but PSA also rises as a man's prostate enlarges—either naturally, with aging, or as a result of BPH (benign prostatic hyperplasia) or prostatitis. A doctor can determine who has BPH or prostatitis and who has prostate cancer by following up a PSA test of 3 or higher with a biopsy. (Overall, only about 30 percent of all men with an elevated PSA will test positive for cancer.)

Is there such a thing as a "normal" PSA that is applicable to any man? Not exactly. "Normal" depends on the age of the man in question. From fifty to fifty-nine, normal is 2.5 or less; from sixty to sixty-nine, it rises to 4.5; and between seventy and seventy-nine, 6.5 is considered normal.

There is some controversy surrounding the use of the test. The objections most often raised to routine screening are that:

1. Detection does not always mean saving lives.
2. False positives may occur when the PSA level is elevated but cancer is not actually present.
3. False negatives may occur when the PSA level is in the normal range, even though prostate cancer is actually present.
4. Routine PSA screening is costly.

How quickly a man's PSA rises—called PSA *velocity*—can be more significant than the number itself. And for those who have *already* been treated for or diagnosed with prostate cancer, PSA screening is the most reliable tool at this time for observation; more important, after treatment, PSA is an essential tool for monitoring the success of the cure.

Some researchers have suggested that men might benefit from earlier PSA testing—at age forty instead of fifty, to establish a baseline. Most doctors who utilize PSA currently recommend that screening begin at age fifty, unless there is a history of prostate cancer in the family, in which case screening may begin at forty.

A PRACTICAL GUIDE

SOME TIPS FOR THE MONTH
FOLLOWING DIAGNOSIS

• *If the cancer has not metastasized,* or if it is contained within the prostate, there is plenty of time for research. Encourage your partner to read up on the various treatment options, and discuss them as knowledgeably as you can with your doctor. Although technical data are often confusing, if you read and discuss together, you can puzzle it out.

• *The knowledge of cancer is disturbing,* even when a patient is assured that the odds are well in his favor. Never underestimate what this knowledge can do to both of you. Regardless of which treatment option he eventually chooses, you are entering a scary new world from opposite doorways: patient and partner. Keep an eye on each other, and understand that you are both affected by this crisis.

• *Get a second and possibly a third opinion.* There are still, as there were for us, three main treatment strategies, although cryogenic treatments can be called a fourth, and a fifth (HIFU) is on the horizon (see Appendix A). The main strategies include:

• Prostatectomy: removal of the prostate
• Brachytherapy: radioactive seed implantation
• Beam Radiation, which has been supplanted by IMRT,
  a newer, more targeted version of radiation therapy.

"Watchful waiting" (or "active surveillance") is not a treatment strategy per se. Hormone ablation is usually used as a supplement to one of the main treatment protocols, except in older men. For further information, see chapter 5, the Glossary, and the Appendixes.

• *Tell as many people as seems comfortable to you both,* but tell someone! Stoical silence is false heroism. You are not alone, and the only way to know that is by sharing your news with someone.

• *Try to find and join a local support group together,* one that welcomes both women and men. Possibilities: Man to Man, Us TOO, the American Cancer Society. At support group meetings, ask and listen—that's how you'll learn.

• *Go to appointments together,* bring a list of questions, and take notes—or even tape the session. If both of you aren't welcome, then consider getting another doctor, one who understands that prostate cancer is a family matter.

• *Consider carefully the doctor/patient relationship.* Is this doctor open to discussing sexuality? What post-treatment strategies does this urologist recommend for getting urinary and sexual function going? How willing is this doctor to describe the side effects and aftereffects of treatment?

• *Consider psychotherapy or counseling for yourself,* and encourage your partner to consider it, too.

CHAPTER THREE

THE COLD CHAIR:
One Body, Two Lives

A VETERAN INSOMNIAC, Dean often wanders at night. Sometimes he falls asleep in a Deco easy chair in the corner of my study, after a bowl of cereal or a midnight glass of milk. One night in early November that's just what he did, an audiobook for company. Thinly covered, he awoke in the cold hours of early morning. The terrifying knowledge that his body harbored renegade cells had sunk into the deep turf of his sleeping mind.

NOVEMBER

Unwilling travelers on an extended journey, we now had a plan: injections and pills—hormone ablation therapy—to begin right after Key West, in January. Then seeds would be implanted sometime in the spring, an outpatient procedure. Just a year, we thought, of what doctors like to call "discomforts," then life as usual.

That November, Dean looked into the mirror and saw no difference, drew one more healthy breath in an unbroken series. From what he understood, if he accepted the treatments, life might resume as normal, or almost normal; he might even make it to old age.

In truth, he—we—understood no more than the bare language of tests and proposed treatments. Medical jargon, like the few words of a foreign language you get from a phrasebook: PSA, Gleason grade, bone and blood analyses, margins, CT scans. But he had no pain or external symptoms.

After his bone scan the previous month, a sassy hospital lab technician gave him a rough/playful push, "Man, this cancer is no big deal—you just got shot in the butt. It ain't pretty, but you'll be okay." That point of view was not unusual: early-detected prostate cancer is easy, "the curable one."

IN DEAN'S WORDS

I remember settling into the overstuffed chair in the study. I got my bowl of tapioca and a Coke (caffeine and sugar at 1 a.m.? No wonder I had trouble sleeping!). I started to listen to voice mails, then called sports phone, then clicked on whatever recorded mystery I was listening to. After diagnosis, I just couldn't finish anything. I'd listen to the first cassette of a book over and over, forgetting who the characters were, or what turns the plot had taken. *I have cancer. I have cancer.* That night I tried over and over to make sense of this murder mystery, whatever it was. Then I switched it off.

It was cold. The furnace had gone off an hour before. I was almost ready to sleep, but because of my insomnia, I didn't want to risk waking up by going to bed. I took an afghan and tucked my feet up under me. I covered myself up as best I could, but I wasn't really warm enough, or at all comfortable. For the first time since I'd gotten the news, I felt really sorry for myself. Life is not fair: you know this from a very early age—that you have seventy or eighty years, if you're lucky.

That night in the chair, I was thinking, *I'm mostly blind and I have cancer and I'm cold.* I started to cry, and then I must have fallen asleep crying. When I woke up a few hours later, my head was tilted to the side, the tears had gone down the side of my nose and formed a pool right in the side of my mouth. I wiped them away; they were so cold. Light was breaking through. One thing I knew after that night: I'd have to screw up my courage and eventually tell everyone in my life.

We wanted to believe that the whole thing really would be that simple. The military undertones of "shot in the butt," with their careless masculine bravado, seemed admirably tough. But they distracted us from thinking hard or seeking advice, anecdotal or otherwise, about how our lives might change. "Battle," "Hitler" (our term), "shrapnel" (one doctor's joking code for the seeds), even the new "active surveillance" (aka "watchful waiting"): cancer isn't war.

WHAT WE KNOW NOW

Like most road maps, ours failed to show topographical features of the landscape. Who knew those were mountains of doubt, depression, or isolation we'd be traversing in the dark? Or that our marriage would be shaken as we went for stretches alone, each of us? Who knew what the lasting effects of treatment would be? Many couples find that the cancer crisis unites them. It has ultimately had that effect on us. But first . . .

We have had to discover how different we really are, Dean longing not to be dependent, me longing not to be alone. Don't underestimate cancer, however "beatable" the doctors say it is. And don't forget there are two of you, two lives overturned. We had to change, then separate, and six years later we are still in the process of coming back together.

There is no intelligence plotting the violent overthrow of the body, just cellular madness, more and more wrong switches thrown. One martial term does come close to describing what Dean was to suffer after the fact: "shell-shocked." But the idea of surviving cancer is still so new, you don't hear it.

His urologist had warned about mood swings, weight gain from the hormones, and incontinence problems from the seeds. Loss of erectile function? In some men it's temporary, and since the doctor seemed incapable of discussing in depth any volatile male topics, Dean just hoped he would somehow be one of the lucky ones. He was afraid to push the discussion too far in this direction.

"Don't ask/don't tell" is a lousy medical strategy.

WHAT WE KNOW NOW

The notion of an "easy cancer" ignores the terror, humiliation, and ultimate physical losses, barnacles that cling to treatment. Don't belittle your suffering, or let anybody else do it. Your own or your partner's cancer is probably the hardest thing you'll ever experience.

Only about a month of conventional living remained for us, although we didn't know it. How precious that time was, mostly frittered away. Sex had been infrequent for several years, and Dean's terrifying news hadn't acted as an aphrodisiac. Make love? We didn't, much, and we regret it. Counseling together, as we entered treatment's dark waters, might have helped, but nobody recommended it. Add E.D. and loss of libido to tiredness, overwork, and insomnia—so many knots in the post-treatment skein to unravel. Some couples are at peace if they come out on the other side and carefree sex is a memory, but that has never been true for either of us.

Each night we went to sleep pelvis to pelvis. Despite his insomnia, we usually woke where we had started out: me tilted on the left

> ## WHAT WE KNOW NOW
>
> Get a second and possibly a third opinion, I tell the ghost of myself. It will give you comfort and some sense of control, even if you end up going with the original protocols. Choose a doctor with an obvious human dimension, one with whom you can both communicate. Join a support community that serves and welcomes both of you. Talk.

edge of the bed, next to the window that contains each morning the rising sun, and Dean sprawled on the right by the dimmed TV.

After breakfast most mornings, Dean was off to Park Avenue in a town car, while my Volvo wagon crept to Yonkers in early rush hour. Dinner commenced around eight. Dean's appetite was hearty. We ate (still do) each night by candlelight, a light he loves for its diffuseness. Spinach, perhaps sauteed in garlic and oil, crusty bread, tuna with olive butter. We shared wine. He helped me bring in the dry cleaning or the groceries, without getting tired out. Nothing was different. But everything was different, suffused with the light of change.

Soon Hitler would be crawling into his bunker. Wouldn't he?

Thanksgiving. It lies at the bottom of November, persuading us into winter. Our table is usually full, six or more guests happy to eat our traditional meal: wild turkey with black walnut sauce, Dean's beloved stuffing, pumpkin soup, homemade cranberry sauce. But this particular year, everyone in the family seemed to have plans. We felt lonely and a little sad, but greatly relieved. Then our niece Debbie called; so there'd be a pretense at a holiday after all. (Why did we have to pretend?)

Since we couldn't imagine a big table laid for only three, I suggested the Boathouse on Central Park Lake, an elegant setting and good food. We were feeling not a little sorry for ourselves, hardly ready to face winter or to feast. We had hoped to lie low until the end of November, then tell the world one person at a time. We wanted to see Debbie, but didn't want to tell her the news, certainly not on a holiday weekend.

I made a reservation, lucky to get a table near the window at sunset. We'd go to a movie afterward. As it turned out, dinner *was* a movie.

I remember all the colors—maroons, deep umbers, and burnt orange—but not the tastes; service was a bit rushed, and there were plenty of little girls in red velvet dresses. The foyer contained a grand fire in a splendid stone hearth. We spent a lot of time sorting out East Siders and West Siders in our conversation, watching the sun fall into the lake. We were masquerading as our old careless selves.

When I'm terrified, a bright interval—good meal, diverting book, walk along the shore—is what I remember later, not the misery. That meal was probably unexceptional, but it was luscious to look at, and being surrounded by healthy young bodies in a glass house on water, eating the foods of deep autumn, marks the evening now in memory. Not telling seemed easy at first. Debbie was untouched by this thing; why not leave her that way?

The healthy young bodies, ripe tomatoes and corn, the sun in the lake. Dean and I were both aware of the difference: the world going on as usual, while our small lives had changed. Lying always

IN DEAN'S WORDS

I felt like an extra in *Hannah and Her Sisters*. That's what I was, an extra, hired to fill out the crowd in a restaurant scene. Of course, in movies all the actors are fakes, but because this was a real-life movie, I was fake—we were fake—and all those dressed-up little girls and their parents were real, they had a right to be there. Deb had a right to be there, too. It was beautiful, and it should have been fun.

separates. Our news, this knowledge of cancer, was a heavy weight we'd have to lay down soon.

Two people already knew: my friend and the therapist she'd recommended. At first Dean had been angry that I'd told anyone, as if I'd let some terrible spirit out of a jar. My therapist wondered how we'd managed to keep quiet so long. How scared I was—and lonely. I assured her that I knew we would be just fine; I only needed "about five months to get things straight." Six years later, I still see her every Wednesday night. This thing is more complicated than either of us imagined, than seeds, machines, instruments, or shots. What's at stake? A marriage; the whole pattern of daily life.

Dean had no one to talk to apart from me, but he would soon. A number on a Post-it, slipped over the counter by a thoughtful receptionist, may have been the only human thing to come from that urologist's office: a support group was forming, so there would be other men for him to talk to. Eventually, he would meet these men face to face on retreat. Meanwhile, those last days of November, there were sudden new voices "meeting" nightly on the phone, through conference calls and an intricate network of voice mail.

I was glad he had his new community. But what about me? There were support groups, some open to wives or partners. But fear and denial (and, admittedly, poor Internet skills) kept me, for the time, ignorant and lonely.

The night Dean slept in the cold chair, I lay in our bed, under a down comforter, on my right side, clenching my teeth and clutching my body pillow, oblivious as always to his nocturnal wanderings, but not to the forces that were beginning to reshape our daily life together, and our marriage.

YES, YOU CAN FIRE YOUR DOCTOR—
ONE COUPLE'S STORY

We may live in the era of the educated patient, but the trappings of doctoring still engender passivity on the patient's side of the desk. Dean should have fired his first urologist. He didn't discuss the possible, even probable, aftereffects of the treatments he proposed; he never suggested that Dean might want to seek second or third opinions; and, most important, Dean didn't really trust him. He had cancer, so he was afraid—and doctors can be intimidating. Anybody who has ever had to fire someone knows how hard it is; and letting your doctor go can feel like firing your boss!

We never switched, but I spoke with Gloria, who helped her husband, Charlie, to switch urologists. At age fifty-eight, Charlie had a Gleason grade of 7.

How did your husband learn about his cancer?

"He stumbled on this whole thing by accident. He had a torn meniscus that required surgery. As part of the pre-admission testing, they did a PSA, and it came in at 5.3 or 5.4. So after the surgery, they referred him to a urologist who worked out of that same hospital. This urologist was the younger partner of a doctor who had been there a long time. He was not confident, although he was obviously smart. I went with Charlie to the second appointment. By this time he had had an *attempted* biopsy. He had not completed it the first time because the doc was doing it without any kind of anesthesia. Charlie was jumping around so much the doctor said, 'I'm going to have to schedule you for another time when I can get an anesthesiologist in here.' So that's why I definitely went with him for the biopsy that actually happened, the second attempt, because I had to drive him home.

"He was lying on the table waiting to be given something and the anesthesiologist asked, 'Didn't you have one of these before?' And he said, 'No, we never got through it, because I couldn't take it without anesthesia.' Well, this seemed to shock the anesthesiologist, this previous lack of concern for pain, combined with the sense we both had that the urologist didn't seem to believe in himself . . . not confident. Well, you don't want a guy you don't trust cutting into your prostate! That was the beginning of the decision to switch.

"He was just so young and insecure in his presence with us, but there was also this terrible fear that to change doctors might get you into something worse. And so I think that switching was up in the air for a bit, long enough for the urologist to start Charlie on hormone ablation. I believe the rationale was to slow the cancer down, give him time to make up his mind what kind of treatment he wanted. So he got that first Lupron shot, along with the Casodex pills. That night he had a horrible reaction to the shot. He swelled up, and he was sweating. It was two in the morning. I called the doctor's service, and I got the older partner—he was very pissed off at being woken up at two in the morning. I was crying. The doctor was angry, and he said he couldn't help me if we couldn't calm down. It was a bad scene. Charlie's reaction finally subsided—we didn't have to go to the hospital. But we were not pleased, to say the least.

"This business with the anesthesiologist was strike one, and then the reaction to the hormone shot and all that clinical coldness was strike two, and then . . .

"Well, I went in to my boss to tell her, 'I may be out more than usual, because my husband has just been diagnosed with prostate cancer.' And the boss said, 'What's his PSA? What's his Gleason?' Then, 'Who's his doctor?' Then she said, 'Whatever time you need, just take it. Two nights later, the phone rang—it was my boss. She got right to the point. 'I've debated whether to tell you this, but I think you should know that my husband was diagnosed with prostate cancer. He had a 6.2, and the doctor your husband is seeing also started him on hormone ablation.' So, it seemed that this practice was going down this road with everybody.

"My boss told me about a friend of her husband's who's a doctor and had had prostate cancer. He had told my boss's husband to stop going to that doctor, stop the hormone treatments, and told him who to see instead. That was strike three—we actually had another choice.

"Charlie's first reaction was that he felt he was following a path. He'd started something, and now what's the danger in changing?

"So he had an interview with the recommended doctor, and we just loved him. He was sure of himself, he was cheerful, he was glad to see us, he seemed to empathize with what we were going through, he wanted to see us both, he was funny. Humor helps a whole lot. He seemed to know what this was all about, and wanted to do a laparascopic surgery. I guess we would never have gone for a second opinion if Charlie hadn't felt this first doctor was not quite up to it, not compassionate, and if he hadn't had a reaction to Lupron the first time, and if my boss hadn't called me up!"

What's it like firing a doctor?
"I seem to remember that the first doctor tried to tell Charlie he was making a big mistake. Six years later the most important thing is that he's still alive. I think that overall the surgery was a success. It was absolutely the right choice. It's such a delicate operation. I can only imagine the incontinence problems if we had gone with the first guy. Charlie's continence is at about 98 percent six years later. Potency? I'd say about 50 percent. [He uses Viagra with fair success.] That's the biggest problem with us, and we don't talk about it. We talk very openly about everything else."

Do you have any advice to give on the subject of switching doctors?
"I would just say, unless somebody said you're going to die in two weeks—and we both know that doesn't happen with prostate

cancer—absolutely get a second opinion, and any doctor who tells you not to get a second opinion is probably not a doctor you should go to. Every doctor probably secretly resents the idea of a second opinion, but the really good ones want you to feel safe about the decision you're making. They know that you need to do this for yourself."

A PRACTICAL GUIDE

TREATMENT RESEARCH AND SOME
COPING STRATEGIES

• *Join a prostate cancer support group in your area:* Man to Man and Us TOO have chapters throughout the U.S., and most groups these days accept women (see Appendix D). Call the American Cancer Society for verification and for a list of groups in or near your area. *If your partner won't go with you, consider going on your own or starting a group of partners or wives.* Don't underestimate the importance of getting to know other couples or women in the community face to face, voice to voice. Cancer is frightening, and community serves a dual purpose: subduing fear while offering practical information.

• *Online, visit the ListServs* (reading online but not responding, sometimes called "lurking," is just fine). Join in the chat when and if you're moved to do so. A complete list of these online discussion communities is in Appendix D (prostatepointers.org, PCa_Women @yahoogroups.com, and prostatecancerinfolink.ning.com are some prominent ones). There is a collegial quality, a camaraderie, to these sites, although nothing beats face-to-face contact.

• *Find out everything you can about all the major treatment options* (these are discussed in greater depth at the end of chapter 5; also see Appendix A). Discuss everything you learn, with both your partner and his current doctor. Prostate cancer treatment protocols are highly technical, and the comparative data can be confusing, even to health care professionals.

• *Read about and discuss as much as possible the anticipated post-treatment effects.* Temporary, permanent, or partial erectile function and continence have featured prominently in recent reports in the *New York Times,* with emphasis on inadequate or confusing data. These discussions point to the fact that, to date in the United States, there is no single treatment method guaranteed to preserve both continence and erectile function *as they are.* Doctors are often reluctant to admit how much treatment may alter a man's (and, by implication, a couple's) life in years to come. Medicine tends to concentrate on "putting out the fire," not on quality of life within the house afterward. For some older couples, incontinence, loss of libido, or erectile dysfunction may not be as difficult to accept as for couples in their fifties. "Quality of life" issues are different for every person, results are different for every cancer, and statistics are different for every treatment option.

• *Will your partner be subjected to hormone ablation therapy?* This is the systematic elimination of testosterone production, discussed in chapter 6 (also see Appendixes A and B). Follow the discourse on this topic at various ListServs, and be aware of its implications for possible effects on libido. To date, its effects are still underplayed. In discussions of sexuality, the mechanics of erection still tend to get all the attention. Viagra, Cialis, and similar drugs are mechanical—they do not affect libido.

• *Consider your love life in its current phase.* Despite how terrifying cancer is, now is the time to talk to your partner about your sex life (and by all means take time to be intimate, in whatever way seems natural to you). The psychologist Abraham Maslow, who posited the famous hierarchy of needs, would probably say that when life is threatened, other needs take a backseat. True, but post-treatment, you and your partner will want some kind of physical intimacy. How can you preserve or enhance physical pleasure?

What is your partner's definition of *intimacy*; does it rely on erectile "performance"? Therapy or counseling could be helpful now, or later. *Doctors unwilling to respond to you about this issue are not doing their job.*

• *Consider psychotherapy for yourself, and urge your partner to consider it as well.* Each of you is entering this crisis from a different direction. Cancer is like a house with front and back doors. Each perspective is different. Couples counseling may also be in order.

• *Tell someone—if not everyone—in your life.* The people you tell may know other patients and partners with stories you'll want to hear. By remaining silent, you are robbing yourself of community and information. There is nothing brave or strong about total silence. Whom you or your partner choose to tell is a personal choice.

• *Do something just for yourself each day if possible, starting now.* You may find this to be your toughest assignment! The hardest thing for those of us who find ourselves cast in the role of "caregiver" is to think selfishly. Time is often the hardest thing to grant yourself, but it's so important to do.

And then what will you do with it? Go walking on the beach. Take yourself out to lunch, with a friend or alone. Get a massage. Swim. Garden. Take a luxurious bath. Your husband's cancer is happening to you, too, and chances are you're not getting much attention or consolation right now. Take care of yourself; there's a reason why the FAA requires air passengers to put the oxygen mask on themselves before putting it on someone else. What good are you to the people who depend on you if you're in a state of collapse?

CHAPTER FOUR

KEY WEST REPRIEVE:
After the Doctor's Waiting Room

Harboring a cancer without symptoms . . . I had
the sense of leading a double life.

—Stewart Justman, *Seeds of Mortality: The Public
and Private Worlds of Cancer*

DECEMBER

IT SEEMED MORE important than ever to preserve the peace of the
holidays and our winter vacation. We always begin December making cookies from an old family recipe for Lebkuchen, the ginger-
bread-like dough rolled in sheets, baked and glazed, which we send
in tins all over the country. We usually end it in Key West at a lovely
old hotel between Christmas and New Year's, that brief period
when the New York business world actually slows down. Dean
insisted that he needed a rest, time to reflect; after Key West, around
January 10, hormone ablation shots would begin.

There was a slight risk in holding out for this vacation before
treatment: that he might be the one man in ten whose prostate cancer will grow quickly. We didn't know those statistics back then, perhaps because we didn't want to hear. His procrastination for mental
health reasons was a last chance to make love the natural way.
Beneath our ignorance and denial, we both sensed it. We didn't talk
about sex, though, and we should have.

Key West and Christmas still to come, we lost ourselves with
unusual ferocity to the making and mailing of the annual
Lebkuchen. Buckwheat honey, brown sugar, a pound of butter,

51

IN DEAN'S WORDS

It was surreal, that December, it was like swimming through gelatin, going through the motions of things. My business was in trouble, and the previous summer I'd been approached by someone who wanted to buy me out. So, in the middle of so much change, I added more change. I was told that the treatments I was pursuing had a 97 percent rate of success for cancer contained within the prostate, but what would life be like after? I made a bargain with God: take potency if you have to, but please don't leave me incontinent.

I regret that bargain now.

brandy, cloves, cinnamon, twenty cups of sifted flour, a tablespoon of baking soda in a cup of hot water, six eggs, walnuts, almonds, citron, candied orange peel. As always, we got the giant bowl down from the high shelf, then boiled the wet ingredients and sifted the dry, cracked the eggs into a bowl and beat them. Dean took, as he always does, the long-handled wooden spoon with the big paddle end, and so began another Christmas. He stirred, I added wet to dry, until the huge dough was finally blended. Let it sit at least twenty-four hours, then roll it out into great sheets, cut the sheets into small rectangles, and bake pan after pan. Glaze with lemon frosting, and the next day pack the cookies into a couple of dozen tins collected over the year from secondhand stores.

As I sealed the tins that fraught December, I recognized ones I'd bought at a Connecticut junk store back in July. Blessedly ignorant I'd been then. There was a shiver that year that went directly into the tins with the cookies; I wondered if any of our family and friends would feel it.

By this time we had told them all. My sister had come up from Philly, the first to get our news. She'd been shocked, as people always are when the word *cancer* enters the conversation. The tone of the conversation changes. You never know how the listener will respond: look away or look down? The etiquette and the grammar of mortality. Later Judy admitted she'd been just a little angry that we'd held out so long. We told the others in a series of phone calls: the Cincinnati base of both families, a niece in Chicago, a nephew in Germany.

There was a polite distance in these brief conversations, sympathy combined with fear. Dean's was the first cancer to be reported in my immediate family—until then, only aunts and cousins had tested positive, most after finding a lump, and all had died within a year or two. For all its treatability, cancer remains scary, slippery, a truth it's hard to hold on to or to swallow. One friend I confided in seemed embarrassed, then quickly changed the subject.

Dean told the rest of his staff and some close friends the week after Thanksgiving. Several old business cronies would drift away on receiving this news—find excuses not to return his phone calls, too busy for lunch, and so on. So it goes with cancer, as it does, no doubt, with AIDS. Susan Sontag in *Illness as Metaphor* reflects on the isolation of patients whose diseases are (or used to be considered) incurable: leprosy, TB, cancer, AIDS. My nickname for this social avoidance is *leprosy thinking*.

In mid-month Dean met the radiation oncologist who would plan and supervise the "planting of the seeds" in his prostate. He already knew about the alternative treatments—excision and external beam radiation—but asked about them anyway. "From all the statistics I'd had quoted at me," he recalls, "the seeds appeared to offer the greatest chance for normal recovery; it seemed the least invasive approach."

"Least invasive" is a splitting of hairs. At the crossroads of the male body, there is no noninvasive treatment. And the seeds were only half the proposed protocols; the effects of the other half, hormone ablation, had been understated.

I sat in the reception area trying and failing to read a magazine with several of the pages ripped out. Light snow was falling outside

53

IN DEAN'S WORDS

If I hadn't been scared before I met the radiation oncologist, I was now. The last wish I had that this could all be just a terrifying dream died right there in his office. It was a sumptuous place, high ceilings and dark, carved paneling. I left Vicki in the waiting room beneath a huge chandelier. Then off I went: it was like meeting a celebrity backstage. First a series of interviews in different rooms, culminating in the brief appearance of the doctor. I knew I hadn't been granted much time with this brilliant fellow. I felt it was important to start the discussion myself: "What are my options, Doctor?" He reminded me of Hawkeye Pierce from *M*A*S*H**: dry wit, tough but a little tender. He picked up a pen and put it down. I could just make out the movement, the gleam of the instrument. He gave a brief gloss of the alternative treatments, excision and external beam radiation.

"We have three possibilities: burn it out, cut it out, or you die."

"That's easy," I said, trying hard to chuckle. "I'll take one of the first two."

the terrace doors in this office, which seemed like a ballroom. Medicine, like so much else in New York, is at times just one more thing for sale, another kind of merchandise with, in this case, all the fantastical trappings of class and privilege. We were supposed to be impressed, and we were. This doctor wasn't on our plan, but after the deductible had been met, the better part of his fee would be paid. It seemed we'd be getting our money's worth.

I stared into the cut-glass gems of the ancient chandelier and wondered what it would take to get the kind of support I needed to survive this crisis. A few nights before, after Dean had been on the phone a long time with his support group, I'd asked hopefully, "Do any of the wives and partners of the men in your group want to form a circle of support?" He promised to ask. But his answer the following night had been an emphatic *no*: no names were to be shared outside the group. They had signed a statement protecting each other's anonymity. Then the shocker: the men "just don't want to talk about their wives, since some are married to women who seem to be walking out."

Who were these deserting wives? A fair number of them, it seemed, were much younger than their husbands. Perhaps these women couldn't imagine dealing with all this messy midlife cancer. As a result of hormone ablation, many men were already going through weight gain, hot flashes, and the like. Younger women, I imagined, might be unwilling to accept a life with likely challenges to spontaneous sex. Later, I would read Karen Propp's moving memoir *In Sickness and in Health*. She was in her early thirties and her husband forty-three at diagnosis, but they'd stuck it out and even conceived and raised a child between the first and second positive biopsies.

I'd already begun poking around on my own for other partners to talk to. One evening while Dean was away on business, my Internet fumblings landed me at a porn site. Rage, then tears. Another time I stumbled into Circle of Love, a community (still in existence today) devoted to wives and partners of men with prostate cancer. Wasn't this, finally, what I was looking for? But the Internet is still oddly distancing to me, even when I chat with people I've known for years. Perusing the site, I'd felt strangely unmoved by the poems and inspirational testimony. At the time it seemed somehow too cheerful.

Searching for community is so personal; it depends on taste and inclination—and timing. My Internet literacy was so rudimentary, I wouldn't have known how to find the appropriate chat rooms or health site boards, though some did exist then. If I had it to do over again, I'd do what it took me four years to do: attend the monthly meetings of our local support group, even if that meant being the only woman in the room.

So there I am, the long-ago me, as in a glass paperweight: waiting for my husband, getting what warmth I could from the chandelier's icy fire, seeing snow falling all around. I turn as Dean emerges tentatively from behind one of several closed doors. We flee the elegance for a watered-down Coke and a lukewarm cup of tea in the hospital cafeteria.

A worker was moving tables and chairs on a heavy cart from one end of the cavernous room to the other. Each time the wheels of the cart hit another floor tile—*thwuck*—the end of one of our sentences fell right through that crack into the floor.

"This doctor's the best in the city," Dean reassured himself, by way of telling me. We talked to encourage each other. The seeds would be "planted" in spring, just as the last of my lettuce was coming up in the backyard. Before that could happen, the regimen of hormone ablation would virtually eliminate testosterone production, beginning in January. *Hormone* comes from the Greek, "setting in motion." *Ablate* is from the Latin, "to carry away." The very term speaks to the degree of change that is likely in a vital fifty-five-year-old man. And speaking of terminology, there's always the charming medical slang we didn't know then but that would have certainly made the procedure hit home: "chemical castration."

The first scheduled weekend retreat of Dean's group, the men he chatted with nightly on the phone, happened shortly after the appointment with the radiation oncologist. Since members came from communities as far away as Portland and Los Angeles, these actual meetings over the months of winter and spring would be few, usually in dormitories on campuses near major cities: Boston, Chicago, San Francisco. Physical proximity would add a new dimension to these friendships and some considerable comfort, faces Dean could finally put with the voices he'd come to know: "I felt isolated before, but included afterwards—part of something, finally: a community."

I was glad he had these men to talk to. But there was no way to reach him in that long-ago Boston dorm room; cell phones and

Internet usage were forbidden. This was a serious retreat. He could call in once on Saturday or Sunday, standing in line to use the pay phone. I respected the cloistering, but I felt entirely alone, and I wondered about the effect of cutting these men off from the communities that contained them. Meanwhile, I was cloistered, too, against my will: a wife inadvertently abandoned by the system set up to strengthen her husband. This model is flawed. Not only does it leave out the other sufferer, but might not the presence of a few women have helped some of the imperiled marriages?

Man to Man, in both the chapters I've visited, welcomes women: the membership is strengthened by our presence. I joined alone, four years after the fact, and Dean eventually came to sit beside me. But that dismal winter, all we could think of was getting away.

Key West, the calm before. *Vacation* is a peculiar word, with its cousin, *vacant*—the sense that nobody's home. We were pulling out of our old life, ahead of a slow-moving managed wall of fire. Despite what lay ahead, we were determined to have a good time in Key West. We'd sleep late, then sip giant glasses of fresh orange juice on the terrace in the clear sun, watching the teal horizon, the catamarans and shrimp boats beneath their odd trapezoidal sails. Me with my laptop and a series of books, stuff I never read anywhere else: *Best Science Writing of 2002* and other heady material. Dean with an entire duffel of audiobooks. My daily swims, his walks to and from the airport. On account of his limited vision, Key West is the only place he feels comfortable walking for exercise. The sidewalks are so smooth and flat, there is no likelihood of his tripping over an unnoticed crack. And with the sea to his right, walking the edge of the island, he never has to worry about intersections. Not that he doesn't negotiate some of the most difficult intersections in the world every day, but on vacation he wants to do what the fully sighted world does every day: just walk.

At Land's End, as far south as you can go within U.S. borders, we slept late for twelve blessed days, the warm wind from the sea fill-ing the sheers at our open terrace door. I remember this as a last time of sleeping together innocently. We would return to this very room the following year a changed pair, but for now we cuddled and made love, oblivious.

For years after, I would wake crying, wondering, was that it? With testosterone nearly zero and libido somehow dormant, our love life was to become a strange new world. Some men sail through hormone ablation with few difficulties. Others may feel uprooted, depressed, or angry. It took four long years for the burning in his penis, from scarring caused by seed implantation, to subside enough for Dean to say, "I miss desire." Healing is like mourning. Burned tissues, depleted gland, enraged psyche, confused sense of who I am, who I was. It can take years and, for us, it has. If we'd gone for joint counseling, the healing might have begun sooner. But it's never, ever too late.

IN DEAN'S WORDS

I usually love the thrill of win-or-lose, but I remember that winter, starting in December, as a time of avoidance. If I thought a team I rooted for was going to lose, I'd turn it off in advance. That game just after New Year's had already gone into overtime once: Miami vs. Ohio State. I was watching on the TV in our room. You could hear them down at the hotel bar, all those Miami fans. When it seemed as though my team, Ohio State, couldn't pull it out, I just hit the power switch: I couldn't stand to watch. It was after midnight anyhow. Turns out Ohio State had won, and I'd been too scared they'd lose to risk watching the end.

During that vacation, everything seemed the same, the light strafing the water brilliantly as it always does at the southernmost tip of Florida in December, but something had happened to us, or was about to happen. It was slow going, this change. You could feel the weight of it, but you couldn't see it yet. It had all started in the oncologist's waiting room, with the questions we were both afraid to ask. It ended as we cried our way to the tiny Key West airport with its innocent prop planes taking off just a few feet outside the door to the seedy Conch Flyer bar. One by one, each flight took its turn clearing the scrub oaks on its way to Miami and Fort Lauderdale, where sad travelers caught bigger planes north to the blizzards of New York or Boston or Chicago. I was staying on for a few days at a writers' conference I had already paid for, reluctant, but assured by Dean that the first hormone ablation shot would be "no big deal."

It would prove to be a very big deal after all: reducing his body's vital juice, testosterone, to near zero production. "Zero T," our nickname for this therapy's goal, would always seem cold as a bone-chilling January day to me, despite Dean's inevitable hot flashes. It had been a month of fire and ice, from the crystals of the oncologist's chandelier and the snow outside his windows to Key West and back again.

A HEALTHY CONSULTATION

Not long ago, I had the privilege of sitting in on a consultation a urologist conducted with a patient and his wife, who were shopping for both a doctor and a treatment. The tone was generally friendly, and I was impressed with how often the doctor brought mild (and entirely appropriate) humor into the conversation. Indeed, given my own personal experience, I was surprised that the couple seemed so relaxed with this doctor that they had agreed readily to allow me to sit in. I felt comfortable enough toward the end of the meeting to speak, when asked to, about my own experiences as the wife of a man who had been treated in recent years.

The woman was taking notes, and her husband seemed comfortable with that. She asked most of the questions, and he seemed relieved not to have to. The doctor's welcoming tone and his broad approach to treatment made for an informative and comfortable conversation (under such circumstances).

The patient was sixty-five years old (Gleason 6, stage T1c, PSA 10) and had been recently diagnosed. The doctor began by asking the couple what they knew of the various treatment methods. Indeed, the wife had done quite a lot of research. They seemed inclined toward the seeds, but definitely interested in hearing about all the options.

In a friendly manner, the doctor proceeded to describe in lay terms the main variations of radiation and prostatectomy. (See "A Crash Course in Current Treatment Options" in Appendix A.)

I thought, as he talked, about Dean's appointment with his radiation oncologist, who said he could "burn it out or cut it out." This doctor was saying basically the same thing, but in far gentler terms. What a difference.

"What about the seeds?" the wife queried, her pen at the ready.

"You're right at the edge of the radiation years," the doctor observed to the patient; "that's sixty-five and beyond. Below sixty-five, I like to incline more toward surgery, assuming good heart health and other factors. The seeds are one of two possible applications of radiation; why would you want to use up this option if you don't have to? If your husband uses radiation—either seeds or beam—first and the cancer returns, then prostatectomy is difficult or impossible to do." Prostatectomies as Plan B are often unsuccessful because the delicate, previously irradiated tissue of the adjacent bladder naturally creates complications.

Toward the end of the appointment, the hard-scribbling wife looked over the top of her glasses and asked, "Tell me, Doctor, if my husband were your brother, what would you recommend?" The doctor paused briefly. "I would recommend a prostatectomy, all things being identical." What a great question to ask, and the right moment to ask it.

A PRACTICAL GUIDE

QUESTIONS TO ASK THE DOCTOR

A tape recorder or notebook should have accompanied you so far throughout the process of settling on a course of treatment. Assuming you have investigated—together—the treatment options (which will vary depending on age, size—of the patient and of the prostate—Gleason grade, PSA, margins, sensitivity to radiation, and yes, lifestyle), you are ready to move on to treatment choice. Presumably, unlike us, you have gotten several opinions; that is, you have not allowed yourselves to be led passively to a single "recommended" treatment plan without examining all treatment options.

Following is a list of questions to ask the surgeon or radiation oncologist. You will surely think of more.

• If the doctor has recommended a particular treatment, then a good question might be, *Why have you recommended this form of treatment over another?* If radiation is recommended, either external beam/IMRT or seeds or combined, then why *not* prostatectomy? If prostatectomy has been recommended, then why *not* a radiation-based treatment? Make the doctor defend the proposed treatment protocol.

• *What are the known long-term recurrence statistics for the proposed treatment, as opposed to other treatments?*

• *If there is a recurrence of cancer, what will the options be for "salvage" treatments?* One of the major disadvantages of any radiation-based treatment is that prostatectomy is difficult, if not impos-

62

sible, as a secondary, or salvage, treatment following recurrence, whereas radiation can follow prostatectomy.

• If the cancer has gone outside the prostate wall, lifestyle may have to go on a back burner. If margins are good, however, it might be interesting to ask, *Could the treatment be matched to my occupation or activities?* If the patient is young and vital, statistics for preservation of erectile function are more promising with prostatectomy than with any form of radiation, regardless of how "noninvasive" radiation seems. A much older man may choose simply to watch and wait, as prostate cancer usually proceeds slowly. Men over the age of seventy may be told they'll die of something else if the cancer goes untreated. Someone who does heavy lifting may choose radiation, as prostatectomy weakens the abdominal wall.

• *What are the possible temporary or permanent side effects of this treatment?*

• If hormone ablation treatments (which virtually eliminate testosterone production in the body) have been proposed, it is sensible to ask, *Are they absolutely necessary and, if so, why?* Some 14 percent of men receiving these treatments find that their libido is low or nonexistent in the aftermath. Other side effects may include E.D. itself, weight gain, depression, and lethargy. (See Appendix B.)

• Additionally, if hormone ablation is proposed, ask, *How long will the course of injections and pills last?* If over six months, questions concerning heart function are in order. Indeed, if the patient has cardiology issues, hormone ablation, which can compromise heart function, may be seen in a different light.

• *What about quality of life after treatment?* What aftereffects of treatment can I/we expect to deal with? The two biggest losses usually have to do with continence and/or erectile function. So a good question might be . . .

• *How can we prepare together for the emotional toll of the changes you have mentioned that might occur?* Is there a professional you would recommend who will work with us to preserve or reinstate, if possible, erectile function? Do you recommend counseling of any kind, individually or together? What books or other literature may be helpful in adjusting to life after treatment, or the hazards to intimacy? *Intimacy,* by the way, is a word you both should feel comfortable using with the doctor(s) who will treat your partner.

In a general sense, there must be trust and confidence among the three of you: doctor, patient, and partner. You, the partner, are part of what is happening, and you should feel welcome. Beware of doctor embarrassment in the face of questions having to do with erectile function or intimacy. These issues are part of the landscape that will be altered as a result of treatment, and they must be addressed.

CHAPTER FIVE

TREATMENT MONSTER OF MANY HEADS:
Sorting It All Out

When a Sick Man leaves all for Nature to do,
he hazards much.
When he leaves all for the Doctor to do,
he hazards more.

—From the definition of *hazard,*
The New Shorter Oxford English Dictionary

THE NEW YEAR found us trapped in our limited view of what was possible or even likely, and ignorant of the aftermath of Dean's chosen treatment. Our choice was a rush to judgment, a grasping at first remedies offered, with faint attempts (on my part) to understand what the implications were for survival and recovery, physical and emotional, for both patient and partner. We could have done better.

This is not to say, looking back, that we made the wrong choice. A letter dated October 16, 2007, from the office of Dean's current urologist, states: "I just wanted to let you know that your PSA is undetectable, and everything looks fine." A blessing: *undetectable.* What better news could a man five years out expect to receive? Well, that erectile function and libido are fully restored, yes, because it's human to hope for more; and that he can drop the regimen of drugs he still takes to regulate urinary surges and flow. But all this pales before the question of what to do if cancer returns.

Was it the right choice? Is there such a thing? The wise choice? Perhaps not. It was a partially informed choice, which left us unprepared for treatment consequences and less well defended in the face of any recurrence. A man as young as fifty-six with a Gleason of 6, stage T1c (PSA at time of treatment 12.8), *might* have been better advised to consider nerve-sparing prostatectomy. These days, he might even be asked to consider "active surveillance," although Dean could never have lived on treatment's edge in that way. Getting back to prostatectomy, he wouldn't have had to undergo the Lupron injections to shrink his prostate in preparation for seed implantation, so his libido (which still has not recovered) might have been spared. Most important of all, we now know that you can always do radiation later, if necessary, as I've mentioned, but that the reverse is not always possible.

HOW TO SHOP FOR TREATMENTS

The other day, I ran across a hypothetical interview on an excellent Internet site (www.rcog.com), a "demo" model of a consultation. How I wish we had somehow stumbled into this doctor's office! The patient begins by asking the doctor if he should go for some form of radiation. The doctor tells the patient:

> Most men who have prostate cancer immediately focus on treatment. *That is a big mistake.* Right now, forget about treatment. First, understand prostate cancer—about the meaning of PSA, Gleason grade, stage . . . how to determine cure and cure rates for prostate cancer. *Learn about the disease first and then let treatment outcome (cure and complication rates) determine your treatment decision.*

Forget about treatment? For a moment and for the sake of understanding, yes. Nobody ever gave us that advice. The doctors Dean consulted were too busy pushing their own points of view.

The patient, sixty-four years old, added:

> My wife and I have never been more scared. The urologist wants to do a radical prostatectomy. Another urologist said I should have my prostate gland frozen by cryosurgery. A radiation doctor [radiation oncologist] said I should be treated with . . . radiation using IMRT and not surgery, while still another radiation doctor [radiation

oncologist] said I should have a seed implant. A third oncologist said that everybody else was wrong and I should have high-dose-rate radiation (HDR). Each of these doctors claims he is an expert and his treatment method is the best. I am . . . scared and confused about the best treatment . . . . What should I do?

And the doctor's response:

Your experience is fairly typical of what men find when they are newly diagnosed . . . . Doctors typically recommend only the treatment they themselves give. A urologist will talk about surgery and a radiation oncologist about radiation. It can be like buying a car. If you go to a Chevrolet dealer, the talk will be about Chevrolets, and a Ford dealer will talk only about Fords.

That advice is right on the mark. Nearly six years later, how I wish we'd had this doctor's sound advice. While there is no guaranteed right treatment choice, there are inappropriate choices and lots and lots of confusion, with medical egos and reputations mixed in. So many men, like Dean, buy the first "car" they're shown, unlike the "patient" in this model interview, who did go for more than one opinion! Good for him.

In my early ventures through the cancer shelf at the bookstore, I had something like this patient's fear—in my case, a spinning sensation. It was the treatment medusa, many-headed and frightening to behold, who froze me in horror. The books that I glanced at, with their charts and diagrams, statistics and terminology, were overwhelming. Then, because I had a husband who had made up his mind early in the process, my research went no further. Doctors had assured Dean he had made the best choice. It seemed the simplest thing to buy the Chevy from the Chevy salesman and get it all over with. It was all so confusing, so frightening. And because we were, like the patient in the Internet interview, really scared, we went for the quick fix, no second opinions.

Let that not happen to you.

KNOW THE PITFALLS OF
TREATMENT IN ADVANCE

As the doctor in the interview points out, you should learn about the disease first and forget for a moment about treatment options. When you have refined your understanding of prostate cancer—what the prostate is and does, what the statistics for survival are—then try to penetrate some of the language: PSA, Gleason, staging, and so on. Now you're ready to investigate treatment options: cure and complication rates, which treatment might be likely to be most effective given such factors as age, size of prostate, even lifestyle. Yes! Because prostate cancer usually moves at glacial speed, you have this luxury.

How to understand it all? How to choose? All the treatments offered here are current, but technology being what it is, who knows what will supplant this list in time? For now and the foreseeable future, we still have, as when Dean was wrestling with treatment, two

IN DEAN'S WORDS

When my primary care physician first noticed an increase in my PSA (until then, coming as I do from a radio background, I thought PSA stood for "Public Service Announcement"!). Six months later, my PSA was up again markedly. I don't recall the number. I can't see to write most things down, so my memory routinely discards old data. At this point, he suggested I schedule an appointment with a urologist. "If the worst comes to pass," he said (and explained exactly what the worst could be), "you'll want to see this doctor."

My decision about treatment wasn't so much rushed as *tumbled* into over a period of two years.

Circumstance—my fear of abdominal surgery, the privilege of being a patient of a famous doctor (who was also a doctor to the famous)—should not drive a decision as important as this. Good, solid thinking should. I am someone who takes pride in being decisive, who has been organizing or running things from my first Kool-Aid stand, to the high school newspaper and the college radio station and a film company, to several corporate communications departments, and finally a private communications company. And yet, I didn't run my own treatment decision! I had completely bought the package that brachytherapy was the "best" treatment a man in his fifties could get.

I don't want to abrogate responsibility here: I'm responsible. "Let the buyer beware" is the law of the marketplace. I just want to be clear about how, through passivity and medical faddism, you can fall into what only feels like your decision but is really a nondecision—something that will affect the rest of your life.

main options—surgery and radiation—with lots of variations. Understand them before you choose one. *If you skip any material in this book, make sure it's not the Crash Course in Current Treatment Options, on page 155!*

January seemed to go on for years. Dean received his first injection of Lupron and filled his prescription for Casodex, these combined treatments comprising the "hormone blockade" that would shrink his prostate to a targetable size and drastically alter his libido. A certain sluggishness and depression set in quickly, a kind of internal weather to match what we came to call "serial blizzards," the terrible winter of the hormones.

SOME HYPOTHETICAL PROFILES OF
PATIENTS WITH A DECISION TO MAKE

What follows are a few fictitious case histories. They form a kind of template demonstrating how each patient and partner might work in league with an understanding and astute urologist to come up with a plan that's likely to yield the best possible outcome, taking quality of life into consideration. Note that all the choices are from the most established treatment protocols to date: brachytherapy, IMRT/external beam radiation, prostatectomy, hormone ablation, and active surveillance. Cryo techniques do not yet have an established track record for outcomes over time, and HIFU is not yet approved in the United States. (See the Glossary.) *Reserving radiation for a back-up choice in case of recurrence, if the patient is young enough and healthy enough to undergo prostatectomy, deserves consideration.*

1. A man 67 years of age with cardiac problems, who has recently undergone bypass surgery, with a Gleason grade of 6, a PSA of 12, stage T1a, prostate size 90 grams. Treatment chosen: External beam radiation.
   Note: *Cardiac problems and risk of total incontinence for a man of 67 caused the urologist to recommend against prostatectomy; cardiac problems also eliminate the use of hormone ablation to shrink his enlarged prostate.*

2. A man of 61 with Gleason grade of 9, PSA 6.5, stage T1c. Treatment chosen: Six months of hormone ablation followed by brachytherapy and external beam radiation.
   Note: *The Gleason of 9 is extremely high, with the possibility that the cancer has not remained in the prostate capsule.*

3. A man of 45 with a Gleason grade of 6, PSA of 3.2, stage T1c. Treatment chosen: Radical prostatectomy.

Note: *His Gleason of 6 is generally low, but this man is still quite young; prostatectomy offers him the best chance for a healthy forty years.*

4. A man of 64, a marathon runner, with a Gleason grade of 6, PSA of 5.0, stage T1c.
Treatment chosen: Brachytherapy.
Note: *He could have logically chosen either prostatectomy or radiation (he is on the edge of the "radiation years"), but he opted for the seeds.*

Perhaps the greatest difficulty in selecting a treatment for prostate cancer is that so much of what a patient hears from friends and family is already anecdotal. People vary tremendously in what they will tolerate with good grace; reactions vary from individual to individual. "Uncle Troy had the seeds and he seems happy." Or "Joe is back from California after getting proton treatments, and he thinks that's the best thing going."

Even if the outcome is total loss of erectile function or continence, there are men who are content because this means they will be around to cuddle their grandchildren. Are older men easier to please when it comes to erectile function? Not necessarily: there are men in their seventies raging at lost libido or erectile function or continence. Read Philip Roth's *Exit Ghost* to understand how high the sap can still rise (or the memory of it, at least) in a very old tree.

A great deal depends on temperament, lifestyle, and thousands of small but irritatingly important factors (such as Dean's blindness, which had already made him struggle all his life against a perceived loss of power). Then there are categorical considerations: how old you are, whether you have any or all the consolations that aging often brings: an understanding partner, grandchildren, a life that doesn't require daily trips to an office.

That said, to the reader: good luck and Godspeed.

CHAPTER SIX

HORMONES:
How Different Will Different Be?

JANUARY: SHUTTING DOWN TESTOSTERONE

WINTER IN THE NORTHEAST often has a mysterious way of seeming years long. From December 1 to Christmas goes quickly, but after the holidays, time itself can seem as frozen as the ground. For us, that winter was among the worst, a sullen off-white, the color of a wall that badly needs painting. Cancer, it seemed, had laid a hand on the weather: blizzard after blizzard, with ice beneath everything.

During the first week of January, treatments began in earnest: shots (Lupron) to suppress the prostate's testosterone production, given with a long needle once a month, directly into the thigh or buttock, supplemented by daily oral doses of Casodex, to keep the adrenals from supplying supplementary testosterone.

Hormones are prime movers. Ask any woman who has sat through a business meeting with hot flashes, longing to strip away her wool suit. A man whose testosterone production has been abruptly curtailed is like that woman, but without a lifetime of preparation for "the change." His default hormone is being taken away against all nature, often with no counseling or emotional preparation. He may have been trained to suppress (unmanly) feelings of rage or fear, to undergo this stripping of what the culture defines as his essence with the stoicism of a soldier.

WHAT WE KNOW NOW

How different a man will be after hormone ablation depends on age and other mitigating circumstances. Had Dean been retired and in his seventies, had he been less mercurial in temperament, had he not suffered from near blindness his whole life, a difficult passage might have been less so. Still, hormones are hormones: the juice of life, the chemistry of who we are.

For the first injection, which Dean assured me would be "no big deal," I am ashamed to say I wasn't in town. With Dean's encouragement, I had stayed behind in Florida for four more days to attend a writers' conference. This decision is a permanent blot on my moral ledger. Dean wanted to go for the shots all alone, and I simply let him. Today, knowing how much change was in store, and how quickly, I would have been on that plane.

Changes, indeed, were rapid. About three weeks after the first injection, the hot flashes set in and sexuality seemed to vanish. Dean showed mood swings and depression, too, and a new feeling of remoteness.

We probably saved a good deal on heat that winter, as I went through the last of menopause and he went through his impromptu change of life: his and her hot flashes! I opened the window on my side of the room just as he closed his. He also had violent mood

IN DEAN'S WORDS

I should have been more scared. Being strong was the worst thing I did to myself. That first injection, I bled a lot. But the bleeding didn't hurt as much as what I knew the doctor was doing to me, to my vital juices.

swings. He once cried bitterly when the spinach he'd sautéed for us burned and stuck to the bottom of our best skillet. Slammed doors were almost routine.

And on top of all this, we had to deal with Cheeno. When we fetched him from the kennel after the Key West trip, our frosty-muzzled old Lab mix was skeletal. I knew the moment I saw him that twenty-one days, even under the expert care of a fine vet, had been too much for this dog, who'd been staggering and falling down since July. He was sixteen years old, a centenarian by dog standards. A rich chocolate brown, he still had that froth of white on his chest—and so his name, Cappuccino. Over the years, the hairs on his chin and his "eyebrows" had gained a dusting of white, all the more charming, but he was much more gaunt than he had been the month before; now he had the aspect of a ghost dog.

IN DEAN'S WORDS

"Please God, don't let Cheeno die now." I said this looking up at the gray sun. Here was this withered animal who would have been dead three years before if not for steroids, and I was asking a divine power I don't believe in, "Don't let him die—not now, not this winter." I think now if only I'd carried him all the way down those iced steps each time he had to go outside . . . but I was tired and it was so very cold.

FEBRUARY: THE HORMONES ARE TALKING

Many people hate February, but for me it almost always contains great hope. Even beyond the fact that it's the month of my birthday, budding branches, Valentine hearts, the ridiculous myth of the groundhog, there is usually a lightness. But that year was an exception. There seemed little chance of spring anytime soon. Had there been no cancer, no Casodex, no Lupron, no dying dog, no mood

IN DEAN'S WORDS

Cheeno represented so much. I'd been forty-one when he was a puppy, carrying stones home in his mouth. I still thought of myself as young then, continuing into my fifties. My youth died with him, absolutely. As for the cancer, I do think I was going through a variation on the Kübler-Ross stages. Denial: this isn't happening to me. Bargaining: Cheeno isn't going to die. I'm not going to die. Anger: I hadn't let myself know how scared I really was. All of this—the diagnosis, the treatment—had taken so long to happen. It had been almost a year between the two autopsies—I mean the *biopsies!* I can't afford that kind of slip.

swings, the month still would have seemed brutal. There was a perpetual glaze of ice on the back steps, the wind seemed insatiable. Wind, weather, keeping an old dog alive; these things masked a greater despair. It was what the hormones were doing, and the great unknown of seed implantation we had to contend with.

Early that month, Dean's support group met for another weekend retreat, at a naval base somewhere in Maryland. A few of the guys were ready for seed implantation, while others were, as Dean

WHAT WE KNOW NOW

I do believe the patient and partner or family should not have to ask for counseling; it should be built in, especially where hormone ablation is concerned. Until it is, there is the Internet, including a variety of ListServs, the American Cancer Society, Man to Man, and more and more books. Physician assistants are another resource. Don't go it alone: you don't have to.

was, still receiving hormone injections and pills. All of these men got hormones in advance of seed implantation. All complained of some combination of the classic side effects: depression, nausea, hot flashes, weight gain, loss of libido, and lethargy. (For a complete list and discussion, see Appendix B, page 163.) Having a group of fellow sufferers to gripe to, and with, when faced with a bizarre treatment regimen may have saved Dean's life. There are stories we hear from time to time of lonely suicides, men who embarked on the protocols without any real support. That January and February, he was grateful for his group. I was grateful for it too, just lonely.

If I had found some women, any women, to talk to, I might have felt less lonely. I later found that some chapters of Man to Man and Us TOO welcome women. But that winter I felt Dean was "covered" with his group, and used to tell myself, "You're not the patient." Years later, when the American Cancer Society Web site welcomed me as a cancer survivor, I burst into tears! So much for solitary heroism. I was keeping a journal and that, for the time, seems to have preserved my mental health.

We were still sharing a bed, but the sea wind off the porch, always loud in winter, and insomnia often drove Dean downstairs for a late-night conference call with some of the guys in the group who couldn't sleep, either.

Just as Dean walked the hallways at night, getting a snack or plugging in to the nightly telephone conferences of his group, down at the vet's, Cheeno—who now lived there during the week—had the run of the place. One morning, reviewing the closed-circuit tape, the vet's assistant observed that Cheeno had kept walking nearly all night long—around and around the examining table in the center of the room, our ghost dog, dragging his lame left haunch as he went. He made it all the way through February, beyond my unremarkable fifty-fifth birthday, this brave spirit of youth who spent only the weekends at home.

I was training teachers in the Bronx and Yonkers that year, the endless drama of urban public schools that thankfully kept me diverted from Dean's moodiness and the ordeal of watching testosterone levels plummet. It was "part-time" work but, like all teaching, filled more hours than were technically required: the planning, the commutation. Up at 4 a.m. three mornings a week to cross the George Washington Bridge before it closed to single-occupancy vehicles, I often napped in my parked car in Riverdale. Once I'd arrived, I was grateful to be of use to the teachers, to be away from the drama of a dying dog and the unpredictability of a husband who seemed to need more and more time alone, waiting for his prostate to shrink. We were both looking forward to the seeds in May. We expected that to be the easy part.

WHAT WE KNOW NOW

If Dean had had a prostatectomy, it would have been over by then—there's a prime argument for surgery! And no hormones! Six weeks, then back to work. But in a period of economic uncertainty, would his business have survived? How many health care decisions are career-, finance-, or insurance-based? These are the toughest decisions of all, balancing health and daily life. Ironically, it's the younger man, who can best withstand surgery, and the older, retired man, with plenty of time on his hands, who is often advised to have seeds, beam radiation, or hormone blockade by itself.

By the end of February, Dean's mood swings had become severe. Who was this man I faced across the table? I was living with someone who seemed to be a combination of a teenage boy and a perimenopausal woman. Rarely, I'd think, "good conversation, good food, this is fun!" He'd make a similar observation, then say with surprise and regret, "Oh, I forgot my pill." The hot flashes, the rage, minute dilemmas blown into great detail. I cleared the plates and glasses after dinner—usually his job. If I did everything, he felt guilty ("You shouldn't have to do it all"), but he was too tired to do much himself; generally he just shrugged and shuffled off. What was so clearly, and sadly, missing was his sense of humor, his greatest natural gift.

I began to teach myself how to discriminate between Dean and the hormones. When he fell into the dark sea again, filled with despair or confusion, I'd remind him, "The hormones are talking!" and we both could laugh. Occasionally he'd stop in mid-rant and make that observation himself. Humor got us through—it gave us perspective. In retrospect, I find this to have been an essential survival tactic. Dark humor it may have been, but that is what we needed.

Just how much the hormones had changed the tone of things was hard to define, perhaps impossible for Dean to perceive at all. In *Hit Below the Belt,* which I read later that summer, Ralph Berberich, who endured both hormones and seeds, observes, "I had no idea that I was depressed. . . . I continued to smile at work and at home, I thought. I socialized with others, continued to visit my aged mother, ate dinner, watched TV, read books. It was at home that my partner pointed out to me, sometimes in jest and other times in earnest, that my verbal response to almost anything tended to be pessimistic."

Dean's mercurial temperament had sent him into psychotherapy in his middle years, to deal with anger at a difficult upbringing and his roughly 96 percent blindness. He had moved beyond this anger years ago, but now it seemed we were moving backward in time, peeling away layers of an old wound. Once, therapy had taught him to level his responses to crisis and lower his stress, to ask for what he needed, and to understand his anger at blindness. His need for self-sufficiency (which he cannot sustain because of blindness) had nearly split us up a couple of times. Now it seemed we were right back where we started, eighteen years of growth and maturity erased in a couple of months. I can still hear him: "I don't KNOW what I want . . . just leave me alone!!" So I would fly into the kitchen muttering, crying, and plunge a few pots into the gray suds. In a very large house, it seemed there was barely enough space to contain us both that month.

Bad as it was in our household, with a dying, incontinent dog and unending snowstorms, many of the men Dean had come to know were alone. By this time, more than a few were divorced or separated. For how many were these mood swings steeped in loneliness? Eating all their meals alone, some men were gaining weight, as predicted.

Weight gain: this was a problem we'd never had to deal with. Because we love to cook and on account of my obsession with finding the freshest local ingredients, we eat healthy, varied meals. These months of hormone therapy were no different. There are very few cans on our shelves, and our freezer is filled with single-portion leftovers—no packaged dinners. Many of the men Dean had come to know who lived alone ate cheap fast food as a matter of course. Often, they treated themselves to an extra order of fries or a dessert after a quarter-pounder, the depression (and loneliness?) encouraging them to overindulge.

Still, by the end of February, I wondered if we were coming unmarried. After years of waking and sleeping together in the same bed, depression and sexual lethargy were working against any kind of physical intimacy. Add to that our sleep rhythms, which have always been at odds: the insomniac and the easy sleeper, the early riser and the late-nighter. His nocturnal challenge with hormones (exacerbated later by seed implantation) became sleeping at all. If I lobbied for a few minutes' reading in bed, the light kept him awake and he'd be up the whole night. Before treatment, these conflicts had played themselves out quietly and been suppressed in compromise, but his moodiness and physical exhaustion and my growing need to have some time for myself at the end of the day sent one or the other of us out of the bedroom for the night sooner or later.

Looking back, in some awful way I needed our coming apart. In tears over what seemed the death of our marriage, I secretly relished time spent in the living room or up in the attic, reading myself to sleep. I needed to be away from his crisis. We humans are not simple creatures. Some nights I spent sleeping on the sofa near Cheeno's "corral," a kind of geriatric dog hospital/playpen we'd constructed in the warmest part of the house. I was keeping him company, this old dog, and we were both staying alive.

MARCH: OLD DOG, OLD FRIEND

Fifteen years before cancer, when Cheeno first opened his golden eyes, there wasn't a gray hair on either of our heads and arthritis was something old folks had. Nobody back then in my household thought about cancer. Back then, Dean could still eat Indian food!

He had character, this old dog. As I held him on his dying day that March, I thought about the arbitrary division between human and animal. We had developed a personality in this creature—stubborn, loyal, devious, affectionate—and now we were losing him by degrees. He was in pain, but unlike some dogs I've nursed into old age, he never snapped at me when I moved him. Cheeno's breathing had suddenly become shallow. We set up an impromptu bed on the dining room table: plastic, blankets, some old pillows. Dean held him and we both thought, "Well, this is it. We won't have to call the doctor." But he was too stubborn; somehow, he fought his way back to us.

The vet was a good friend. Knowing how hard this would be for us, he offered to pay a housecall when the time seemed right. We called him and waited the horrible half-hour for him to come, trying not to cry. We offered Cheeno smoked salmon, a favorite extravagance, but he was beyond food. The doctor came, and it was done quickly.

How to carry something that only a minute before was your friend, fifty pounds, still warm, out of the house to a waiting Jeep? Our vet isn't a big man: he staggered under the weight, so Dean took the burden.

Fifty-seven years old with prostate cancer, taking hormones to shut down his body's production of youthful juices, going through the resultant mood swings and depression, sexuality lost, life itself in question and full of confusion, Dean carried his dead beloved dog down the goddamn frozen back steps one more time.

APRIL: DIAL-A-MATTRESS

Our two souls therefore, which are one,
Though I must go, endure not yet
A breach, but an expansion,
Like gold to aery thinness beat.

—John Donne, *"A Valediction: Forbidding Mourning"*

Dean and I weren't separated by a great distance, like Donne's Renaissance lovers; it was only a few yards from the second floor to the third floor. Still, it was a distance. At night, with no Cheeno to worry about, I found myself climbing those attic stairs, so familiar now.

Dean wanted to be alone. The hormones had made him a wreck; he was confused and frightened, he needed to sleep, he needed to walk the hallways. He needed to talk to his group on the phone. These were long and private conversations; the telephone cord stretched across the hall to the bedroom, our bedroom, and the door was shut. I wanted to come closer, to hold him and to comfort him, but he kept pushing me away. As tales of marriages drift back to me now, marriages that have broken up while men were on hormone therapy, I'm amazed that ours made it through. Save for dark humor, there was little pleasure for us then.

Every couple handles cancer differently, and every treatment protocol is particular to its patient and that patient's situation. Men in their late sixties or beyond whose cancers are particularly slow growing may undergo hormone therapy with fewer of these agonizing side effects. Such a man's testosterone levels may have been low to begin with, and, in any event, he is likely to have been retired for a while and less sexually active than a younger man. But for a man of fifty-six, still active in a competitive business world, the sudden shift away from testosterone can be like a push off a cliff edge.

IN DEAN'S WORDS

First it was plain old insomnia that made me want to sleep alone; later on, it would be urinary "surges" and embarrassment about being incontinent. You don't feel attractive when you have cancer. But at that point, I couldn't exercise; the hormones made me just want to go to bed, and all I wanted was solitude. Little pills, little pills—about the size of an old-fashioned saccharin tablet—are drowning your sex drive, and you fear that you'll lose your edge.

It's hard to distinguish between what you feel and what you think you feel. I couldn't tell the difference between what Casodex did to me and the concept of Casodex. Those few nights when I forgot to take it, I'd sleep better. Was that the hormone? Or the concept of the hormone? Hot flashes, mood swings—I understood why people want to commit suicide. Too much change. I felt like I was sitting next to death. For me, and for so many men, prostate cancer is "mortality lite." With my stats it's usually treatable and you'll survive, I was told, if you take your medicine and go for one of the procedures. But everything in your life is out of control.

As for myself, it was some consolation that I had been exiled to an agreeable setting: two rooms and a bath with the nicest tub in the house. Ultimately, the attic became my refuge, though I kept trying to sleep downstairs with Dean, where I had for so many years. Some time ago, the *New York Times* published an article on couples sleeping apart. I can't say how much it comforted me to learn that even relatively young couples often build houses these days with two master suites! Insomnia, mattress firmness, snoring, and general nocturnal habits, not to mention the tastes and inclinations of two adult human beings, often lead people to move into the guest room or build a new equivalent master suite. I wish I had read that article when we were first getting used to sleeping apart, which we still do about half the time. I wonder how many marriages have broken up because people think that the marriage bed must define the marriage?

So, while Dean's life had taken an oddly adolescent turn—the cord under the bedroom door, the excessive need for privacy—I was having my own teenage reversion. To comfort myself, like a freshman making a dorm nest, I bought some lamps, good towels and sheets. The bed was a problem, an ancient, stained queen-sized mattress on a wooden platform, not easy on a fifty-five-year-old back.

One night over dinner, I complained about it. On impulse we called Dial-a-Mattress. Brilliant! This was a move that may have saved our marriage. That night, in my hypercritical mood, I thought it almost too cheerful. Was Dean trying to buy off the guilt of banishing me? If he was, I think now, it worked!

The mattress man on the phone observed, "A mattress is an important purchase. Think of it as something you'll enjoy the rest of your life." He had no idea I was married and moving out, all under one roof.

The next day it came, my "space mattress," made of a material invented for astronauts that responds to body temperature. Who knew it had marriage-saving properties as well? It was the most expensive queen-size they had in stock, and we ordered it not because of its orthopedic merits (which I now treasure), but because we could fold it to carry it up the corkscrew third-floor stairwell.

There's something a little outrageous about sleeping three stories up, in a room small as a capsule, on the mattress that went into

WHAT WE KNOW NOW

Buy something that is for your body and your body only. Indulgence could take the form of massage or elegant clothes, but in my case, climbing the stairs to sleep on a surface that molds itself around my shape diverted me from the terrifying separation we were going through.

space. That mattress was for me only; it held me as Dean once had, and would again, and it taught me to sleep singly and well, one floor above.

I began to write this book in the relative solitude of the attic. Audrey, our remaining dog, kept me company much of the time, curled on the edge of the new mattress. I'd installed a teapot, rigged up the old stereo, imported a bottle of brandy and some tea biscuits. Beyond my dormer windows, the birds were singing me awake: we had made it, at any rate, through winter, looking into spring. It was seed time.

CHEMICALLY INDUCED ANDROPAUSE: EFFECTS ON PATIENT AND PARTNER

Although there is apparently no documented proof of natural, observable andropause—the age-related decline in serum testosterone, sometimes referred to as PADAM (partial androgen deficiency in aging men)—it would seem to be real for men who have undergone androgen ablation therapies (what else is the virtual absence of testosterone in a man, if not "change of life"?). In a 2003 article in the journal *The Oncologist,* Dr. Charles L. Loprinzi of the Mayo Clinic notes that the concept of andropause in prostate cancer patients is poorly represented in medical literature.

Medical acknowledgment of induced andropause could help some men and their partners recognize physical changes such as loss of muscle mass, breast swelling, loss of libido, fatigue, depression, and the like, enabling them to survive this confusing, disorienting, and often discouraging treatment process. When hot flashes begin and periods become infrequent, we women know what to call it. If these men are to have their sudden change of life, how can we help them weather the crisis?

CHAPTER SEVEN

AT THE HOSPITAL:
Where They Don't Heal, But Save Lives

MAY

SEED TIME: the part we thought would be easy and painless. This surgical procedure was what the months of testosterone deprivation had been leading up to. Dean would be gowned, sedated, and placed on a table in lithotomy position (similar to childbirth) in a hospital operating room. In attendance would be the surgeon, his urologist, a dosimetrist (who calculates the placement of the seeds), nurses and other support staff, and the star of the team—the radiation oncologist, whom Dean wouldn't actually see until his post-treatment consultation a month later.

It was a Tuesday; Dean fully expected to be more or less back to normal on Friday. We had packed our bags and checked into a hotel in midtown, close to the hospital and within a taxi ride of his office.

The hotel we chose was not inexpensive; knowing an ordeal lay ahead, we both looked forward to room service and soft sheets. This is actually a tradition in our family, dating back to my first knee operation, the first of eight arthroscopies—all outpatient, but all involving what doctors call "discomfort" and patients call "pain." Hospitals are not friendly places, generally, and going home, where the dishes may still be in the sink, the trash overflowing, is traumatic for caregiver and patient alike. This we did well: making a careful landing place, post-op.

Another built-in comfort: I'd asked my sister to come up from Philadelphia to keep me company. I think it's smart to take someone to sit with you in the waiting area. The seeds were scheduled for noon, with Dean (so we thought) out of the hospital and on his feet by six or earlier. We'd go back to the hotel and put him to bed. We'd talk and have a light supper and Dean would go to sleep. It all sounded so manageable.

But our lack of anecdotal information, and the casualness of the term *surgical procedure,* as opposed to the more blunt *surgery,* hurt us deeply. We did know of one man who had recently had the seeds and been up and about with minimal pain the following day, and we'd read of others. Optimists that we were, we assumed that would be Dean's outcome as well. We were scantily informed. Since I hadn't been sitting in on consultations with the urologist and radiation oncologist, we had only a sketchy notion of how the seeds would be placed, how Dean would be positioned, even who, exactly, would be head of the team. I have since met several men who have had seed implantation who don't know which kind of seeds are in their bodies or how long they'll be active. One at a Man to Man meeting wanted to know when his low-dose seeds (always permanent) would be removed!

Most important, we did not fully understand how common urinary irritation—burning and scarring—is post-brachytherapy. These symptoms can be permanent, as we know all too well. Dean seems to be among the unlucky 5 percent who will probably spend the rest of their lives taking several drugs to ease the flow of urination and counter irritation. We were certainly not prepared for the severe emotional effects of incontinence. Other side effects having to do with the bowel are definitely attributable to the seeds. The E.D. he has suffered from is attributable both to hormone ablation therapy and to the implanting of the seeds, as all radiation treatments carry with them the danger of scarring.

Of course, back then we didn't know what to expect. We'd been told to be at the hospital at eight a.m., but where? The reception

---

WHAT WE KNOW NOW

Know what you're in for, or likely to be in for. "Let the buyer beware"—*caveat emptor*—goes double for medicine.

---

area we'd been directed to report to had no record of the procedure. They directed us to another waiting area, which redirected us once again. So, at around 8:30, after several false turnings, we found the part of the hospital we were expected to wait in, but there was nowhere to sit. What had once been an office corridor had, for space reasons, been given over to a series of very small waiting rooms. The room we were shown to had six chairs—certainly all that room could contain—but eight people were already in there. Dean stood, and I sat on the floor. Eventually we inherited one chair, which we took turns using for about an hour and a half. Finally, all the other waiting souls had been called away, and we inherited the small provisional waiting room, along with the right to turn off its television: President Bush on the deck of the aircraft carrier, having his "Mission Accomplished" moment. My sister arrived, a little breathless, around 10:30, her train having been stuck in an Amtrak tunnel. Without my cell phone (which wasn't supposed to be on), she might never have found us.

At 12:10, the urologist appeared in scrubs and paper slippers, irritated that his patient wasn't dressed yet for surgery. He and Dean quickly disappeared, then reappeared, two big men in loose, clowny garments. Scared, I kidded Dean—the gown with the little flowers, the paper cap and slippers—then regretted it after he'd vanished into the steel-doored world of the O.R. Apparently, after donning his patient's uniform, Dean was ushered to yet another small waiting room, where a man sat dressed for hand surgery. He was crying, while a woman in street clothes tried to comfort him. Dean had no one to sit with, no audiobook to listen to. There were no magazines—not that he could have read them anyhow. Why had the doctor sent him away to sit alone in his thin cotton gown—open, of course, at the back—while other patients, apparently, could still keep company? My sister and I were a corridor away.

What would I have done without her that day? A nurse told us where the family waiting room was and advised us to get lunch right away, so we'd be ready and waiting when the procedure commenced. I remembered how to find the cafeteria from our visit with the oncologist.

We slid our trays past the glass shelves and exited with salad, tepid coffee, and the fried chicken one nurse had told us was "just like Mama's" (it wasn't). The daily ritual in that airplane hangar of an eatery hadn't changed since our visit four months before: the dragging of heavy cartloads of chairs from one end of the cafeteria to the other over the tile floor—*thwuck,* interval, *thwuck*—still made conversation unthinkable. We were hardly tempted to linger; at least in the waiting room we could talk.

But it wasn't a room. In fact, just as the "waiting rooms" we'd sat in initially were really former offices, this new space was really a mezzanine overlooking a central atrium. Although there were plenty of comfortable sofas and the inevitable television, this space had been designed as a pass-through, a place to pause and look down on foot traffic.

As it turned out, the hospital was preparing for a medical conference that evening, and the atrium was being transformed into a meeting room. Was any space in this hospital *not* makeshift? Hospitals everywhere have to struggle to survive, and this one was no exception, packed to the gills and using every inch of its public spaces for purposes the architect had never intended. These days I resent it all fully and openly, as I was too frightened to do back then.

My sister and I were at least treated to a bit of Fellini. Beyond the railing of the mezzanine (for us, just at eye level), workmen on scaffolds hoisted great illuminated spheres—like weather balloons—above what would be the conference floor. Men and women with clipboards paced the gleaming marble floors efficiently, barking orders for the placement of each sphere, each table, and the dais. A man with headphones tested the audio: plenty of feedback. Down there everything seemed to be floating, dreamy, and hardly quiet. The coffee wagon normally available in the atrium, the one consolation we could have been offered, was closed.

In our balcony lounge, we sat with other families, each waiting for a particular bit of news from an older woman who sat with a telephone and files at a large oak desk. There were others: a young Hispanic family and a Sephardic group of five, which included a rabbi pacing up and down, talking on a cell phone. He wore a black silk tunic with about two dozen tiny, closely set buttons up the front and what appeared to be opera pumps. You notice these kinds of details when you're waiting for someone in surgery. One or two people looked tense, about to burst into tears. The woman at the desk was kindly, but severe. She cautioned each party not to leave at the same time for coffee, in case a doctor might call. She meant well and she knew what she was doing, but I still felt sent back to third grade.

Just as we had closed down the first waiting room, we were among the last to leave our mezzanine. The woman at the desk, our link to the world, was apparently a volunteer, due to leave at 5:30. She conferred on us and the Hispanic family, her last two charges, responsibility for each other. It was now up to us to answer the phone.

Around six the urologist, still in paper shoes and scrubs, materialized. The procedure had been a success: 107 seeds (iodine-125) had been implanted, and the patient was resting in recovery. With a half-life of sixty days, these titanium seeds, about the size of a grain of rice and coated with iodine-125, would slowly release radiation to the areas of Dean's prostate that were known to harbor cancer. But where should we go to find Dean? The doctor seemed irritated at such a question (to which he didn't know the answer) and vanished as quickly as he had appeared, like a paper genie.

Logic sent us back to the cramped corridor where our day had begun; it was, of course, the nurses who led us to Dean, sitting up in a wheelchair, still in his flowered hospital gown. It was late by this time, around seven-thirty. A little group of nurses had gathered around my naturally funny husband, who, despite sedation, was proving he could still hold court. When could he leave? Not until he urinated independently, which he passionately desired to do. A small assortment of beverages—apple juice, water, even a a cup of tea, which he despises—stood on the tray next to the wheelchair.

On her way out, the head nurse presented us with a one-page document on hospital stationery stating all the things Dean should be careful to do or not to do:

- Wear a condom during sexual relations for the first two months after the procedure *(ironic in retrospect)*.
- Children should not sit on your lap for more than five minutes each day for six months *(after an iodine-125, which Dean had had, but just two months after a palladium-103, which has a much shorter half-life and, along with cesium, has now more or less supplanted iodine-125)*.
- Remain at least six feet away from a pregnant woman *(for three months after an iodine-125, one month after palladium-103)*.
- Touching, shaking hands with, or kissing a pregnant woman is permissible.

We could sleep together, apparently. Where was the pamphlet on "Your Life After Brachytherapy," with helpful tips for couples? Where, for that matter, was the urologist?

It was late. Dean still hadn't urinated, and everyone, nurses included, wanted to go home. Coke being what the patient longed for, an orderly took my sister and me on a quick backstage tour of the closed-down hospital, through a couple of vacant OR's and down some long corridors in search of a vending machine—what a day of theater! Finally, at about 8:45, Coke consumed and urination accomplished, Dean dressed in baggy pants, and a taxi took us to our hotel. Sounds of the conference echoed in the hallways as we made our way down the stairs. I thought ruefully of what a surgeon had told me after an emergency appendectomy: "Go home now; we don't heal here, just save lives." We were going back to our temporary home, the hotel, the seeds of our summer and fall finally planted. As iodine-125, now implanted in Dean's still very large prostate, is only 50 percent depleted at sixty days, it was going to be a long, hot summer. Healing in the full sense would take years.

I had assumed we would share the king-sized bed in our hotel suite, but as it turned out, I slept on the sofa (I'd given my sister the other bed). If Dean had been adolescently shy before, his need for solitude now was enormous. Standing ready on the dressing table, seemingly doubled by the mirror, was his arsenal of medications: Casodex (his continued hormone ablation pill), Cipro for infection, Pyridium for urinary discomfort, Flomax for urinary flow, and Vicodin for severe pain, just in case.

Here was another crossing over: the time of muffled screaming had begun, screams I would overhear in the months to come

---

WHAT WE KNOW NOW

What had been missing was the narrative between doctor and patient, part of the pre- and post-surgical experience. When details come out in retrospect, they can be devastating. The urologist's lack of candor, like stress applied to glass, cracked the relationship, which would end for good a few months later. Easy to say "it's all available on the Internet," which this stuff is, nowadays, but a startling number of patients don't feel comfortable doing their own research or don't have access to the Net or both. They rely on their doctors to be at least somewhat candid about the quality-of-life issues surrounding a seed-placement procedure.

WHAT WE KNOW NOW

"There is little discomfort after the implant, except for some mild soreness in the perineal area lasting one to two days. Mild rectal bleeding or spotting [from the insertion of the ultrasound probe in the rectum] may occur for about 24 hours in the area in which the needles were inserted. There may be a small amount of blood in the urine. This is normal and should stop in one to two days. Your doctor may instruct you to use an antibiotic cream on the surgical site for a few days following surgery."

What would these words have meant to us then? I found this reassuring text easily the other day, with a couple of keystrokes and the search words "Brachytherapy prostate cancer postsurgical." It is certainly easier than it was five years ago to find information, but still not easy enough. Such a text should be part of an official nationwide pamphlet handed to each brachytherapy patient pre-op. Surely, knowing what to expect post-op is as important as knowing to keep your distance from infants and pregnant women.

through a number of bathroom doors. This elegant old bathroom was to be the first. Dean's a big man, strong, but he bruises easily. This time something beyond the flesh had been bruised. Not really trusting his doctor—who seemed to demand silence, compliance, stoicism, and isolation—Dean had not known what to expect during or after seed placement, and neither had I. It had been an assault on his body, as all surgical procedures are. We were only now beginning to understand its effects.

The morning after, Dean laid the phone on his pillow and looked at me, stunned. He was bleeding from the rectum, a post-op development no one had prepared him for (unusual, but hardly rare). On the phone, his urologist told Dean that most of his discomfort had to do with the delicacy of placement. The seeds are inserted via the perineum, the tissue between the scrotum and the rectum. If he had been told these details, Dean had somehow not comprehended them at all; having sat with the doctor alone, he may not have taken in all the salient details. Now he was trying to cope with the rawness, the "discomfort" of post-op. His doctor, sounding rushed, simply assured Dean that there was nothing to be alarmed about.

After two days and a few stolen moments with my sister, we packed our bags, our medicines, diapers, and surgical pads, and went home. Dean had hoped by Friday to be ready for an afternoon at work, but while he'd been prepared for the fact of incontinence (I'd bought diapers and pads in advance), humiliation was another thing altogether. These reactions vary from one man to the next, but as a population, men are less prepared for leakage of any kind than women are. It is possible that, because most urologists are men, the silence surrounding leakage issues is exacerbated. Dean was up six or more times a night to urinate, and there was never any guarantee whether he'd make it to the toilet in time.

There were so many things to deal with at once, all strange. The hormones had already altered his sense of who he was. Now his pelvis was warm to the touch. This frightened him. Although the new warmth wasn't painful and he had been deemed safe to sleep with, he didn't want to be touched or held. His body, it seemed, wasn't his body anymore. Home we went, Dean to the sanctuary of his own bed, alone, as I was upstairs in mine.

WAITING ROOM STORIES

What follows are some wives' voices on what waiting during surgery felt like for them.

ANGIE

"I was waiting in a solarium—all light and air and glass. I went with two other people, a friend and a cousin of my husband's. We were told that it might be inoperable, in which case everything would be over very quickly. Everyone was superb. There was a concierge to relay information to the waiting families. It wasn't impersonal at all, but even at that, knowing what I'd been told about what might happen if it were inoperable, every time a doctor walked through I wondered, 'Is this it? Are they going to tell me something?'"

Angie had company, and she was well treated in a beautiful space. Nonetheless, it was agony for her—in the waiting, not knowing what to expect. As it happened, the operation went well. That was some fifteen years ago, with no recurrence.

TAMIKA

"It was a long ordeal, his prostatectomy. I brought plenty of stuff along to read, and people took turns sitting with me: my mom, some of my girlfriends. It was a long way to the hospital. I had to stay overnight at a hotel, and I'm so grateful that some of those same folks, including my mother, took turns staying with me. I didn't feel that anybody in particular was reaching out to me at the hospital, but through mailings, I knew that there would be support there if I had asked for it.

"What would I want for women in this situation? I think if anybody had asked me to come sit in a room with other wives at the hospital while I was waiting through those long hours during the surgery, that might have been a wonderful thing! What if the wives were each offered a phone buddy? My husband had one, you know—they do that for patients."

Tamika has a good point—a roomful of wives waiting through the same exact ordeal might be a good thing. Lucky for her she has such a marvelous support network!

GERALDINE

"I felt so lonely. Even though they told me that he'd be out by noon, the procedure [brachytherapy] started late and there was a backlog, so I waited eight hours. It was a crowded room and I was all alone—nobody could take off work to be with me. I kept wondering what was going on. I wish I'd had the common sense to bring some music to listen to. Everybody else had somebody to talk to. I'll never do that again, go to a hospital waiting room alone. Thank God everything turned out okay. I just want other wives to know how awful it feels to be alone, so they won't end up the way I did, chewing their nails till they're raw."

Nobody should have to wait alone for someone undergoing a surgical procedure. I did it once and I will never forget how frightening it was waiting for Dean's emergency appendectomy, sitting in the obstetrics waiting room, where the surgeon had told me to wait, with happy families trading prospective baby names.

JOSEPHINE

"He opted for robotic surgery. The hospital staff couldn't have been more supportive. I was placed in a special waiting area just for prostate patients' wives and family. I was told that I would be called on the phone throughout the surgery, and I was—three times! First to tell me he had just gone in, then at the midpoint, and finally after his prostate had been removed and he was being sewn up. I had my sister with me—I was glad of that. I felt so supported; that hospital was terrific."

Little things mean a great deal: the special waiting area, the periodic phone calls, the presence of a close family member. If there is such a thing as a good experience waiting during surgery, this is it.

96

A PRACTICAL GUIDE

WHAT TO DO FOR THE PATIENT
AND FOR YOURSELF

There is frequently little or no hospitality in hospitals. Patient and family often have little or no choice which hospital they'll be spending their time in, as a lot depends on doctors, available procedures or equipment, location, or health plan. So how to survive before and during your hospital time? *Do what we didn't do:*

• Be a medical advocate and take charge of the situation. As I have stressed many times, don't go to consultations alone—you may fail to take in important details of surgery or treatment procedures that will affect the way you experience treatment and may affect how you heal afterward.

• *Go for a second and third opinion* and, in your evaluations of various doctors and methods, be sure to note which doctors seem supportive of the idea of a second opinion.

• *Choose, or encourage the patient to choose, the doctor he feels most comfortable with,* and think of that doctor as a treatment partner. Be wary of any doctor who doesn't seem to welcome this kind of relationship.

• *Attend a support group and ask questions* of others who have gone through what you both anticipate experiencing; compare, contrast: age, Gleason grade, PSA, stage, and so on. You can never ask too many questions.

• *Ask the urologist for a list of specifics on what to expect "the day of."* For example, if you're preparing for brachytherapy, ask the doctor to describe the procedure: the team who will be in the OR, the length of time the procedure will be likely to take, what position the patient should expect to be placed in, and where he may experience pain post-op. Keep in mind that "discomfort" is a euphemism for pain!

• *It may not be possible to choose your hospital, but if it is, choose one where you both agree you'll feel comfortable.* Hospitals that specialize in one kind of disease or treatment (joint-disease hospitals, for example) often house "burned-out" staff who are numb to patients' feelings. Big city hospitals can be trying for other reasons, such as overcrowding.

• *Partners: prepare in advance* for the loneliness and possible emotional hazards of the waiting room. Don't go there alone, bring plenty to read (make that light reading!) or listen to, and determine in advance which room/floor you should come to when called. Get food before the procedure begins and/or bring it with you. Be prepared for the shock of "saying goodbye" to your partner pre-op, regardless of how "inconsequential" the procedure is supposed to be.

CHAPTER EIGHT

THE PARTNER'S SIDE OF THE BED:
What Do *You* Need?

JUNE 2003

I'M ON THE examining table, heels in the stirrups. My gynecologist, a woman in her mid-thirties, is doing all the right things: palpating breasts, deftly manipulating the cold steel of the speculum, asking questions. I sometimes think I'm the oldest woman in her practice: I don't see many others in the waiting room who aren't pregnant or at least of childbearing age. I sometimes imagine that she's learning what to say to menopausal women in her conversations with me.

"Active sex life?" she queries with studied ease. There is, probably, no casual way to ask this question, and odds of a sharp retort rise with the age of the patient. "Of course not," I fire back; "my husband has prostate cancer." We make small talk about his treatment regimen: the pills, the injections, the seeds. On the subject of hormone shots, she is more candid than any doctor Dean has consulted so far. "Wicked stuff," she whispers, sadly.

Sexuality is the ultimate "quality of life" issue for cancer survivors. A May 2008 Cancer Care teleconference panel, "Rediscovering Intimacy in Your Relationship Following Treatment," taught me a few things I wish I had known about what was happening to our marriage and quality of life when cancer hit. It would have helped me when Dean was angry and hostile to see his—and my—sexuality as part of our respective identities, not just as a strong physical urge we all have. We were not prepared to have our identities—the "potent" man, the "sensual" woman—changed so suddenly while we were coping with a life-threatening diagnosis. It didn't help at all that Dean's urologist preferred to avoid the topic of sexuality. He's not unusual; many doctors seem embarrassed, or hyper-professional, so they downplay sexual change. Perhaps "chemical castration" threatens some doctors' own ideas of manhood. Add to all the confusion that the culture as a whole is blasted daily by what one panelist described as "unrealistic" images of what many people assume is normal, healthy sexuality. The loss of identity, the loss of pleasure as we had come to know pleasure, the official medical silence on everything but the pragmatics of treatment, and the young, nubile world-as-usual made treatment a dark tunnel we traveled together but somehow alone.

WHAT DID I NEED?

Five years after diagnosis this question is still hard to ask, and even harder to answer. I didn't fully know that cancer, which had happened to Dean's body and mind, had also happened to my mind and—yes, in indirect ways—to my body. Thankfully my body was not in pain, not harboring a cancer or radioactive pellets; but my body is not detached from my mind. I was terrified, just plain lonely, and filled with stress. As time went on, these vulnerabilities often took the form of sexual frustration. This last statement I could never have owned when the treatment process was happening, because in those days all Dean had to say was "I have cancer!" to chasten and silence me. What he probably meant was "I'm scared, I'm lonely, I'm angry." But since he felt he had to have everything under control, he just said, "Good night," and waved, then closed the bedroom door. And so—Good night—I climbed the stairs to bed.

I NEEDED TO FIND OUTLETS FOR MY ANGER,
WHICH KEPT COMPANY WITH MY FEAR

Dean was away; he had sailed out from the shore of health, where I had been left standing, bewildered and afraid. Although he'd been assured and I had read that prostate cancer when detected early is highly treatable, cancer is cancer. We had accepted its presence and were halfway through the cure, but the cure was stranger than we had imagined; its effects were more confounding and terrifying and, for Dean, painful than we had been prepared for.

Partially on account of fear but also because of loneliness, I had a lot of anger. I couldn't admit to it, but I did find ways of letting it out: writing has always been my primary survival tool. Little is said in cancer narratives about anger. It may be the ultimate taboo subject, almost as if expressing it will invite the cancer to grow. Women who express anger, especially if their partners are suffering from cancer, seldom meet encouragement. Why should this be a surprise? "Anger is unseemly in women," a long-ago guidance counselor warned me. Beyond writing, during the treatment period I chose safe times to uncoil my anger: screaming my way home locked in my car, or standing on the rocks in Connecticut at high tide.

WHAT WE KNOW NOW

If you have anger, you had better give it some appropriate ways to express itself. If you ignore it or, worse, deny it, it will grow and be as difficult to excise as a tumor.

Anger has to be lived through, given its due, acknowledged, lest it become an obsession. It may even be, as psychiatrist Sarah Auchincloss suggests, the beginning of closeness. So, through our anger and not in spite of it, Dean and I were trying to reach each other. That summer in a bookstore, I spied a rack of cards bearing quotations. I was struck by one, which I bought and framed: white on black, a circle of words credited to Winston Churchill. Though he's not my favorite historical figure, the little broadside is on my desk to this day: *If you're going through hell, keep going.*

My anger was my hell. I took his advice.

I Needed to Touch

And to be touched: innocently, intimately, spontaneously, to know I was desired, if not in the absolute classic sexual sense, then by way of body-to-body contact for more than a moment standing in the kitchen. And not the ceremonial hug with its kiss hello or good-bye.

In my attic, I had a good supply of books and movies. I bought a reading rack to place across the third-floor bathtub, because I love a bath and I love to read. A certain line of bath oils and Dead Sea salts delighted me, along with the thin, wrinkled silk gown I still occasionally wear to bed. There was a particular set of smooth cotton sheets, really old from washing over and over, that always seemed to take the edge off physical loneliness. Someone years before had given me a little lavender pillow, supposed to soothe the eyes. That summer, I cuddled it obsessively the way, when I was a child, I used to press against a certain plush dog as I went to sleep. (Lavender, I later learned, has been proven to induce sleep more readily than other natural scents.) I became an expert in high-end chocolate—65 percent cocoa butter is still my favorite; I keep some to this day in a jar by the attic bed. The brandy on the dresser was an occasional comfort then. My memory-foam "space" mattress was the closest thing I had to a lover; its loamy warmth got me through a lot of miserable nights. These were my indulgences; they didn't take the place of real physical intimacy, but at least I was paying attention to myself.

I Needed to Be Sexual, Even in the House of Pain

Pleasure, pain: we live always somewhere between the poles. Most of us experience pain as something on the order of a toothache, a migraine, arthritis. It piles up as we age, and we accept what happens to us. Pleasure is pain's gleaming opposite. They live close by, in the same body and often at the same time. One Saturday morning, reading myself awake with Shere Hite's 1984 *Report on Male Sexuality,* I turned on my air conditioner to drown out Dean's cries of pain from the bathroom one flight below and to mask any inadvertent whimpers of my own pleasure. Not without residual guilt do I confess this, but giving him the solitude he needed often required diversionary tactics. That summer I read about the women of Nantucket, whose husbands went to sea for several years at a stretch. Many of them used a nineteenth-century version of a sex toy, to which they gave the euphemistic nickname, "He's away!"

Well, Dean *was* away, and I missed him. Loneliness was physical, in a way it hasn't quite been since. I ached to be held; he found touching or being touched repulsive, part of what one psychologist has referred to as the "damaged goods syndrome." He said not to take it personally, but I did. I was fifty-four. It had been a few years since men had noticed me on a street or at a party. I used to flirt like crazy in certain safe private settings, such as gallery openings, and some of these guys, thank God, flirted back. It helped a lot. I treasured a touch on the shoulder, a social kiss. We don't know everything there is to know about human sexuality, and every situation is unique. Some studies seem to indicate higher levels of testosterone in women who make love to themselves frequently.

"Am I a high-testosterone woman?" I sometimes wondered, as I lay alone in my attic bed. I could conjure up a fantasy easily enough, but felt, beyond loneliness, the lead mantle of guilt. It was difficult to let myself have pleasure in the house of pain. With a husband whose body was a mess of hormones injected and swallowed, who had lost his libido and was suffering reactions to the implantation of radioactive pellets and was on fire every time he urinated, unable to sleep because the urge to urinate came multiple times a night, it wasn't just that there hadn't been any sex, but that even thinking about sex seemed unfair. I learned to ignore this odd form of survivor guilt and help myself. Even in the midst of fear and pain and confusion, perhaps on account of it, I needed to have a good time.

If you can manage it, make love to yourself; who knows your body better than you? Most men, and many women, do it all the time. Take erotic care of yourself, whatever that means to you. Guilt is a useless item. Discard it.

I Needed to Get Out of the House and Away from the Crisis

And so I did—taking writing retreats when I could, or going to stay with a friend overnight. Recently, I confessed to a good friend that I actually took a three-week trip abroad by myself. I cried when the plane took off, and I still feel guilty, but the marriage survived.

I Needed Regular Exercise

And I got it. A walk around the block might have sufficed for some, but for my arthritic knees, swimming has been the prescriptive for well over ten years. My personal mantra is an adaptation of an old cliché: *When the going gets tough, the tough go swimming.* I kept up my regimen of two to three sessions a week all the way through the treatment year. I was not doing the kind of active cancer caregiving many partners do, which would have added even more excuses to my list of reasons to skip it. But because I didn't talk myself out of swimming, I was more able to be of use to Dean, which brings me to the next point.

WHAT WE KNOW NOW

Many people whose lives are more encumbered than mine was still manage to give themselves time and space apart: going out to a movie or to a café with a book, seeing a friend, getting a workout at the gym. Do it if you can, and if you can't, just go for a walk around the block.

WHAT WE KNOW NOW

You need exercise, and because of the cancer that has entered your household, which is terrifying, exhausting, and depressing, you need it more than ever. It is always tempting to talk yourself out of your exercise routine: you're tired, there are bills to pay, meals to cook, special vitamins to procure, prescriptions to pick up. But make yourself do it. Exercise elevates your metabolism and wards off disease; it keeps your middle-aged body from going to fat, which, especially in the abdomen, is dangerous. If you keep your heart rate elevated at its exercise target rate, a release of endorphins may give you a lovely natural high. That is probably why I sometimes limp dejectedly into the health club and stride optimistically out. Long-distance runners are, as a population, seldom depressed!

I NEEDED TO BE OF USE

I may, ultimately, have been more useful than I give myself credit for being. Because Dean wanted to be alone, I *felt* useless much of the time, and those feelings no doubt contributed to my own depression. In the larger sense—by keeping the house up and running, dealing with a dog's death and other disasters unrelated to cancer that cropped up that year, fielding questions from friends and family—I was very helpful; and because of Dean's visual handicap, I routinely do many things he might otherwise do himself. It's a shame I didn't see how helpful I really was; it might have improved my outlook. There are many other women—I read their posts on the Internet all the time—who have just the opposite problem: up to their nostrils in caregiving. They probably fantasize about being more useless. Perhaps there is no perfect balance!

I Needed to Understand What
Was Happening to Us

Dean's new loathing of his body and mine startled me. Was this what zero testosterone had wrought? Perhaps in 1969 I hadn't read *The Second Sex* deeply enough. Now I returned to that book and delved into other writings more specifically focused on how men and women differ in hard wiring, how they think about or achieve pleasure, both with one another and alone. The trunk to the left of my bed was stacked with Kinsey, Hite, Foucault, de Beauvoir, Freud, Deborah Blum's *Sex on the Brain*, Susan Bordo's *The Male Body*.

Was Dean, I wondered, clinically depressed? Some 20 percent of all cancer patients may suffer from clinical depression, either as a result of treatment or, in the case of people whose cancer has already presented itself as tumors, from a possible chemical link to depression. Occasional thoughts of suicide, insomnia (increased since the treatments had begun—a side effect, apparently, of hormone ablation), and sudden loss of appetite are all symptoms of clinical depression—and all things that Dean had struggled with while the protocols were going on. Fortunately, his psychotherapist gave him the professional support he needed to keep going.

Meanwhile, as a result of all my reading, I began to write about what was happening to us, and that helped me most of all. When I'm writing, I'm talking to an "other"—the computer screen or the page—and so I am not alone. Then, by some alchemy the voice of the page returns to me someone entirely different, born of my own character.

I Needed to Talk to Someone

And so I had psychotherapy once a week, a strong bond, stronger now than ever. The writing group out of which this book sprang, which meets only every other month, was another lifeline. I brought them chapters; they read and reacted. I am grateful for their careful reading, their compassion—and their astonishment! Other people, people who had no husband with cancer, could read and be

WHAT WE KNOW NOW

I read anything I could get my hands on that was well enough written: novels, history, cookbooks, memoir, and always poetry. All these different books helped buffer the reading about sexuality I really wanted to do. Painful as this reading occasionally was, it helped me, and I know I'm not alone in this. Descriptive posts on topics such as penile implants, libido, erotic fantasy, even the Kama Sutra, crop up all the time on Internet sites dedicated to talking about the effects of prostate cancer treatment. These sites exist for consolation and a kind of solidarity, not to mention information exchange. Many partners and patients need to talk frankly to each other about what has happened to their lives and their marriages.

shocked by what was happening to the two of us. This readership of four made all the difference to me. My older writing group, the group of poets I went to Montana with while Dean was getting his news, helped me in another way, in our biweekly meetings and sharing of poems. I seldom talked to these women about Dean's illness, because I wanted to inhabit an arena where poetry was the focus and cancer didn't exist at all.

There were a few relevant Web sites, but "inspirational" writings have always left me unmoved, and six years ago that is all I found there. But go to ListServs and other sites dedicated to prostate cancer discussion and see what you find that suits your needs. These things are quite individual.

During treatment, as I have discussed, Dean had had his own community, which met almost nightly on the phone; that had left me pretty much out of the loop. Four years after diagnosis, long after Dean's group had disbanded, I finally went to a local meeting of Man to Man. Joining alone was one of the most difficult things I have ever done, and one of the best. Before going to the local group, I fortified myself by visiting (as a researcher) the Poughkeepsie chapter, which spawned Side by Side, a women's support group. Both locally and upstate in Poughkeepsie, I found that the men were grateful for my presence; they welcomed a woman alone!

Recently, a friend and colleague, Elaine Albert—nurse, trained group facilitator, and breast cancer survivor—has joined with me in founding a local support group for partners of cancer survivors, What About Me?, under the aegis of the American Cancer Society. Although not specifically dedicated to a prostate cancer population, the group has taught me things about myself I didn't know. Listening to the details of other stories is the best way to understand your own. How many times has someone in the group begun to speak of a personal need, then gone off at length on injections, biopsies, chemo, or hair loss? Of course, a personal need of the one standing just to the right of cancer is to talk about the body of the loved one, the body actually in the line of fire. But then, if you're going through hell, it's time to keep on going, and ultimately you will come face to face with what you need at that moment.

Not Everybody Is the Same

Among those who have undergone seed implantation, especially those who haven't had hormones, are many who have maintained some form of erectile function—around 50 percent, if recent statistics can be believed—and some whose libidos were spared or only dampened.

Some patients come through pretty well if libido was spared, working hard to achieve erectile function through injections, pumps, rings, or drugs such as Viagra.

Then there are those men who have entirely lost a desire for sex, but their wives don't miss it. Several years ago in a women's group that met during Man to Man, I heard one woman express relief that sex seemed to be "over." Having already experienced menopause, with its waning estradiol levels, she was happy enough to hold hands and watch movies.

There is no such thing as the classic cancer story, let alone the classic prostate cancer story. That said, I meet myself again and again in the stories other women tell, and then I meet women who say things that astonish me.

WHAT WE KNOW NOW

Support groups are another resource. Man to Man and Us TOO, two national PCa networks, have local chapters in many communities. Some of these chapters welcome spouses, while others do not. Spouses and partners sometimes talk of working up their courage to go to meetings by themselves, without the man whose condition is their motivation for joining. So, to any woman who is afraid, I urge you to go. The hardest thing is walking in the door the first night.

Although Dean and I suffered in solitudes of our own, many couples are brought closer during cancer; they go willingly to every appointment together, and they find that their intimacy actually somehow increases. The men in these stories often want their partners to do the research for them, even to tell them what to decide.

Dean needed to be alone, and he felt he needed to make his own decisions, to be independent of me. At the time he was, quite understandably, too busy coping with cancer to know how isolated I was. He did have his group; they were a great consolation. He was taking care of himself emotionally, and I'm grateful to that community for what it gave him. As for me, I did a great many good things for myself, but I could have done more. For example, I probably should have walked into the local Man to Man meeting by myself during the treatment period, when I badly needed the information and fellowship it affords.

This book is a product of the independence I was forced to build as a result of Dean's crisis. In any crisis, you need to look for ways to learn, ways to keep disaster from becoming tragedy.

Faulkner wrote: "Given a choice between grief and nothing, I'd choose grief." In this book, among other things, we are grieving: for our mistakes, for our silences, for what we have lost. We are also discovering ways we've grown, and rejoicing in the fact that we have survived to heal. It's scary to tell this story, but fortifying—like kicking dirt in the face of the devil.

WHY IT'S SO IMPORTANT TO TAKE
CARE OF BOTH PARTNERS

What's it like to be the partner of a man who has undergone not just cancer, impotence, and erectile dysfunction but a radical hormonal shift that seems to have set another man in his place? In a 2007 study, it was noted that nearly one-third of men diagnosed with prostate cancer in a particular clinic had levels of psychological distress that met criteria for anxiety disorder. Looking back, it seems that Dean could have joined these ranks at the time of his treatment.

But there's more: according to another study, when a couple is dealing with any cancer, a *partner's* psychological distress might drag down the well-being of either person! In the April 2008 issue of *Annals of Behavioral Medicine*, Youngmee Kim noted that "the psychological distress of the female partner seemed to have the greatest effect whether the woman was the breast cancer survivor or the caregiver of a man with prostate cancer." (Dr. Kim is director of Family Studies, American Cancer Society's Behavioral Research Center in Atlanta.)

In other words, in a heterosexual relationship, take care of the woman's psychological needs and you have taken care of both partners! That's two for the price of one!

A PRACTICAL GUIDE

TAKING CARE OF THE CAREGIVER

Some Internet Sources

The Circle (www.prostatepointers.org/circle)
Note: prostate pointers is part of Us TOO, a national network for prostate cancer patients and partners, which also offers PCAI (prostate cancer and intimacy) as well as other online discussion groups.

Cancer Care (www.cancercare.org/tew)
Telephone Education Workshop, ongoing teleconferences at www.cancercare.org/podcasts, an archive of available podcasts of older conferences, including "Rediscovering Intimacy in Your Relationships Following Treatment" (May 13, 2008).

The "New" Prostate Cancer Infolink
(prostatecancerinfolink.net)
News source, community, and blog started by Arnon Krongrad, M.D.

Phoenix5 (www.phoenix5.org)
A site dedicated to prostate cancer survival. Among other things, do not miss "For Companions—Their Problems Are Different" and "A Six-Step Survival Guide for Women."

Free Publications

Facing Forward: When Someone You Love Has Completed Cancer Treatment (U.S. Department of Health and Human Services, National Cancer Institute, 1-800-4-CANCER)

National Prostate Cancer Support Networks

Man to Man

A national network allied with the American Cancer Society, with chapters in many cities. Some chapters welcome women, and some even have allied women's prostate cancer support groups, such as Side by Side (see the American Cancer Society or call 1-800-ACS-2345).

Us TOO

Another major support group network with chapters in many cities. The organizing force behind prostate pointers and The Circle (www.ustoo.org).

CHAPTER NINE

THEY NEVER TOLD US:
Post-treatment Surprises

DEAN HAD BEEN warned about incontinence and temporary urinary pain, but burning often resulting in difficult urination (despite Detrol) and lack of consistent flow (despite Flomax) made the continued hormone therapy, with its attendant depression and lethargy, even harder to bear.

IN DEAN'S WORDS

Each time I urinated was like pissing needles. I would fold a washcloth and bite down on it. The burning in the penis remained for a half-hour afterward. A few times I actually put my penis in ice water to numb it. I'd been told I might have a "temporary burning sensation while urinating." Bullshit. I had extreme burning immediately after surgery, then for some reason, while we were still in the hotel, it stopped for a day or two. After that, though, it was with me, this urinary pain, for a long, long time. And for the first time in my life, I was completely incontinent. It was all really hard for me to get used to.

We women are conditioned to survive the surprises our bodies often present to us, beginning with menstruation and ending with menopause. Power, for many men, is linked to issues of containment: of bodily fluids, of pain. And that Dean had already dealt, all his life, with near blindness, made these treatment surprises even harder to bear.

In *The Heroics of Falling Apart,* a breast cancer memoir, Judy Gordon writes: "Falling apart was what I needed to do for myself, but it was hard on others, at least in the beginning. I couldn't be Judy-as-usual. As I went through the process of giving in to my fears, I became unpredictable. Suddenly, I was no longer positive nor upbeat nor optimistic. I had no 'go-for-it spirit' even though I was constantly reading and hearing that [such a] spirit was a requirement."

Dean certainly had lost his "go-for-it spirit," and yet he was still in the business world, still expected to be funny and provocative, the sought-after producer of corporate conferences and his own best salesman. He was certainly expected to contain himself, in all senses of the word.

The summer of 2003 contained another tragedy we hadn't anticipated, which had nothing to do with seeds or hormones but

---

WHAT WE KNOW NOW

Had Dean allowed himself, or been allowed, to "fall apart" for a time, then he might not have been filled with such rage. I wish we had managed to make the time for an ordered collapse, but such a move would probably have played out as his sudden retirement—something we simply couldn't afford. It might even have catapulted us into bankruptcy. Fiscal constraints often color medical experience; they can lead to wrong or hasty decisions, and they can also slow or block healing.

---

seemed to weigh us down even further. Our remaining dog, Audrey, sleek and healthy-looking, was not so healthy after all. She'd had a cyst removed from her anus earlier that winter, and her general unhappiness, I figured, might be a complication of the surgery. The vet started his examination in a chatty good humor, then blanched as he withdrew his hand. What he had found inside her was hard; it would test out a week later as malignant.

"It's not one of the treatable cancers," he told me finally; "it's spindle-cell." At age seven, she was dying from the inside out, although her coat was still glossy and her teeth firm and white. We tried to keep her at least through the Memorial Day weekend, which marks Dean's birthday, but she was so unhappy: bewildered and in a lot of pain. A neighbor who loved this dog almost as much as we did helped carry her in a towel down to the car. The vet was finishing up surgery, so we stood beside the examining table, trying not to cry all over her. What do they sense, animals, when we have made the irrevocable decision? After a while the vet entered the room and did what he had to do. Audrey licked each of us just once as she died.

Now half of what had been our household was dead. A kind of shock settled on us that night as we left the vet. "Where will you go?" the vet wondered. "A very dark bar," I replied, and that was where we ended up. Dinner tasted like ashes. That the cause of this sudden death was cancer unnerved us both. I kept wondering how Dean had managed to hold her during the final injections.

Then the dog dreams began: mine and his. Cheeno walked into his bedroom a few times—*click click,* paws against the bare floor. He'd wake and turn the light on: emptiness. Once he even felt a wet muzzle on the edge of the bed. It was Audrey I saw, dark burning black eyes in a brindled face. These apparitions were, of course, part of the mourning process. But the dog ghosts were something else as well.

The topography of our life had changed significantly in a very short time. Now we lived in different rooms, waving good night like roommates. Meals, once happy occasions, were often interrupted by flights to the bathroom or depressive conversation. Long stretches of Dean's sleepless nights were absorbed in detailed conversations with members of his cancer group. We weren't the people we had been. At this point, we weren't even a couple, and the silence of the household was forbidding. When the dogs came to us, Audrey and Cheeno, in odd moments between sleeping and waking, they seemed like messengers from the old life, the one that had once given us joy and a sense of purpose.

When a pet dies, we never rush to replace the animal. A few months of mourning seem appropriate; after all, these dogs and cats are not commodities or appliances, but living spirits. This time, however, I listened to the suggestions of the vet's receptionist, who had good contacts in the Beagle Rescue movement, and at the end of June we adopted a pair of puppies, George and Gracie, almost a year old. They'd been locked in a garage for six months while their owner was recovering from a heart attack. He'd intended them for hunting, but abandoned them when he realized he would never hunt again. Meanwhile, they had apparently been abused, certainly abandoned, having suffered from a kind of sensory deprivation: fed but never let out, and certainly never loved. They were refugees of a kind, and so were we. It was exhausting training them. Before the summer was out, George had to be put on a kind of tranquilizer. He kept barking obsessively at a particular tree. Gracie threw up, shivering uncontrollably, and her eyes glazed over every time we put her in a cage to transport her. That summer, they were hardly replacements for Cheeno's nobility or Audrey's gentle patience, but they did divert some attention from the quiet hysteria of our overturned marriage.

That summer I realized how misleading isolated pieces of anecdotal material can be when you're trying to prepare for a medical procedure of any kind. Advertisements for seeds or surgery usually stress only the better outcomes; although there are usually valid statistics to support the bragging, there has to be somebody behind the "possible side effects" in small print at the bottom of the page. Brachytherapy, like all treatments for prostate cancer, can differ from patient to patient. Some members of Dean's group had had a much easier time with it. The husband of a friend of a friend had undergone the seed treatment about a week before Dean had. He'd had no testosterone suppression, just the seeds. His radioactive iodine seeds had been identical to Dean's, though perhaps lower in quantity. Back at work the following week apparently pain-free, Larry became a kind of legend to us. How had he managed to shoot 36 holes of golf forty-eight hours after implantation? Gradually, in our conversations, admiration for this man turned to sarcasm: "I heard Larry went rock climbing in Tibet the other day. How *does* he do it?" In truth, the majority of men return to normal activity after seed implantation. Larry's easy course of treatment was at the middle of the statistical curve, and Dean's was at the far end. Unlike Dean, Larry is a small man; his size, and the size of his prostate, allowed the doctor to avoid hormone therapy in advance of seed implantation. So, no moodiness or hot flashes or lost libido. And when implantation time came around, fewer seeds. He may have been an ideal candidate for brachytherapy.

The Casodex, morning and night to suppress testosterone, with back-up monthly shots of Lupron, was one factor separating this robust man from my depressed and pain-ridden husband. Because of Larry's promising example, which had come down to us in a friendly phone conversation the week before seed implantation, we'd had a false sense of how easy this could be. We'd thought it was just a technicality that Larry had had only seeds. But depression, lethargy, E.D., and a general lackluster feeling—the effects, in other words, of the hormone blockade—were like a set of stone weights Dean wore as he swam through that summer.

July seemed dominated by what Dean dubbed "surges"—like "urge," as in "gotta go." In a local restaurant where we'd gone one night for dinner, he excused himself and hurried into the restroom.

WHAT WE KNOW NOW

Try to see beyond the bragging of various doctors or institutions specializing in only one treatment. Ask yourself which set of protocols seems appropriate given the stage of cancer, the Gleason grade, PSA, and whether the cancer is contained within the prostate capsule. The size of the prostate and the age, fitness, and lifestyle of the man in question are all important. What are the statistics for each treatment now, for outcomes and for recurrence? If you select radiation of any kind (which includes the seeds), bear in mind that prostatectomy will not be an option if cancer returns. In other words, try to see the forest for all of those more or less equally sized trees.

Behind that door was an old ventilator, very noisy, but his screaming cut right through the clattering fan. "Could you hear anything?" he queried, back at the table. I hesitated. "I want to know," he pressed; "what if I'm at lunch with a client?" Yes, his howls had been distinguishable, not loud but audible.

He was horrified. Dignity, vanity—these can be significant players in any treatment experience; he had not been prepared for all of this vulnerability. It was hard enough to be incontinent, suddenly wearing pads or actual incontinence pants. But then to have the sudden urge to urinate, often with no success, and when there was success to want to cry out—this is not something a man easily gets used to.

Bleak as some aspects of July may have been, there were others that gave us hope. Slippersilk ears, paws, and gradually widening eyes. What would we have done without George and Gracie? They were our comic relief.

The third consolation was the knowledge that Dean had to live through only three more Lupron shots: the one coming up soon and a double shot in August. The Casodex pills would continue until

November. So, November was our goal. Life as we had always lived it to resume, we hoped, around Thanksgiving—wild turkey with black walnut sauce and a return to normal. But what would this new normal be?

Five years later, we're still finding out.

SCARY STUFF: A WIFE'S-EYE VIEW

From time to time, I read Dean's old medical records. I'm hoping for an increased understanding of dense medical language I was never trained to read, but I'm also looking for something. Why has he suffered so much more than most brachytherapy patients from problems of urinary urgency and flow, and those terrible burning sensations? Five years later, why does he still suffer if he tries to tip-toe away from taking the medicines to relax his bladder and regulate his flow?

Yesterday, I read the hospital report one more time. The morning of implantation, Dean's 90.3-gram prostate had shrunk to only 74.5. In other words, it was still enlarged. Such a prostate, irradiated with seeds, is destined to swell and likely to affect the patient's urination: flow, cramping, you name it. Implanting seeds in a prostate over 60 grams would seem to invite a possible lifetime of urinary complications.

Why didn't anybody question the size of this patient's prostate? Why isn't prostate size one of the things all patients discuss when they discuss a possible course of brachytherapy?

"They never told us" has its flip side: *we never asked.* I never asked. What should a partner who has been discouraged from gathering information do? Gather information. In retrospect, that's what I'm doing by writing this book, long after the fact but with the hope that other people won't make the same irrevocable mistake. If I had done a little more preparatory reading, would I have realized that hormone ablation was more than just, to quote my GYN, "wicked stuff"? Perhaps not. Would I have understood the nuances of prostate size vis-à-vis seed implantation? Not unless someone had explained them clearly to me. I'm just able to grasp these concepts now, after considerable study.

Many doctors push one specific treatment over all others, and the treatment Dean's doctors were pushing was brachytherapy. "One size fits all" frequently means it doesn't fit you.

THINGS A DOCTOR MAY HAVE
FAILED TO MENTION

We are not alone in being surprised by treatment aftereffects; if we were, people visiting prostate cancer Web sites would have a lot less to talk about!

Current wisdom has it (despite what you may hear) that:

- *Nerve-sparing prostatectomy has the best overall survival statistics*—fifteen years out—and the best overall continence statistics.
- *Brachytherapy (unassisted by hormone therapy) has the best erectile function statistics* and the best short-term continence stats, but after about two years, that advantage is lost.
- A recent study reported in the *New England Journal of Medicine* found that *adding hormone therapy was associated with negative outcomes* across multiple quality-of-life domains among patients receiving brachytherapy or radiotherapy. Brachytherapy patients reported urinary irritation, bowel and sexual symptoms, and transient problems with vitality or hormonal function. (The study wasn't explicit about radiotherapy patients' problems.)

If some doctors or institutions claim great success in sparing a particular function—with statistics to back up their claims—some of the success may be due to the way in which that function is defined. A recent controversy has its origins in how doctors (and patients/partners) define the word *erection*.

Drs. Nelson Stone and Richard Stock published a study in *Urology* in 2007 that would seem encouraging for brachytherapy/erectile function outcomes: "Before implantation, 77.2% were able to have an *erection adequate for intercourse* [my emphasis] and 50.6% were able to at the last follow-up visit. A significant correlation was found between potency preservation and age. . . . The preservation of urinary, sexual, and rectal quality of life is excellent at long follow-up for patients implanted with iodine-125. . . . With a minimum of 5 years of follow-up, 61.5% of men with good EF [erectile function] before implantation were able to maintain *erections sufficient for intercourse* [my emphasis]."

What exactly is an "erection adequate for intercourse"? Some men may report partial erections insufficient for penetration, while others are too proud to say how sufficient their erections actually are.

Add to this confusion that surgeons have been known to hand-pick the population of patients they serve, hoping for more successful outcomes. In *How Doctors Think,* Dr. Jerome Groopman observes:

> Failure is something physicians deeply dislike. . . . When I researched outcomes of surgery for prostate cancer . . . surgeons reported a wide range of postoperative impotence and incontinence. Although individual skill of the surgeon may account for some of this variation, as I probed some more it appeared to be largely a function of which patients the surgeon chose to operate on. Some surgeons turned down difficult cases involving large, aggressive cancers. Others refused to operate on patients with serious medical problems, like diabetes, even though surgery was their best option to eradicate the cancer. Such patients are more prone to nerve damage, and thus to impotence.

Finally, men newly diagnosed often act too quickly, picking the first treatment option suggested to them by the first doctor they see (Dean falls into this category). "Research suggests that men who learn they have prostate cancer [often] decide on a treatment quickly, base their decisions on anecdotes or inaccurate impressions, and stick with their decisions even when given scientific information that might cause them to change their minds." ("Prostate Cancer Decisions Often Based on Fallacies," *New York Times,* July 4, 2006).

Why this frequent rush to judgment? Though told that prostate cancer is perhaps the one cancer that affords them time for research, men may panic and pick either some treatment scheme that is still lacking in reliable data or the first treatment modality offered them. Some say they want cancer out of their bodies a.s.a.p. Others are so understandably afraid of the twin perils of E.D. and incontinence that they go for new "miracle cures" with little or no research to back them up. In general, because there is little consistency of opinion in the medical community, the lay community remains confused. (For an excellent description of this phenomenon from the patient's perspective, see Burt Solomon, "In Prostate Cancer Pick a Number, Any Number," *New York Times,* Health, August 26, 2008).

CHAPTER TEN

THE "I" WORDS:

Incontinence, Impotence, Identity

FROM MY JOURNAL, February 2004, almost ten months after seed implantation:

> Snow's erasing the steps outside, the weathervane just above my window is threatening again to veer off toward the harbor. All morning I could hear the phone ringing way downstairs, but writing has become such a compulsion that I never paused. Meanwhile, Dean had something to tell me, calling and calling all morning.
>
> He was at work, and without thinking much about it, he got up from his desk, crossed over to the bathroom, unzipped, and was halfway through before he realized there was no fire. Half the miracle is that this routine act-become-an-ordeal, once so unconscious and pain-free, may be almost back to normal. Are we turning around now? Suddenly, life—and springtime—seem imaginable, long car trips without emergency stops, sleeping in the same bed more often. If he isn't leaping up all the time, then he won't feel self-conscious and will want me to stay through the night. Those moments when he excuses himself, leaves the dinner table—perhaps no cry of pain as he tries to complete this simple, necessary act.
>
> He's full of fresh courage. If we've really reached the turning point, then I should record now, while I remember, the humiliation and the vulnerability.

CONTINENCE: THIS SIMPLE, NECESSARY ACT

Dean's greatest horror was incontinence. This doesn't seem to be true for every man; many guys are more fixated on erectile function from the outset; but the two functions are parallel when it comes to vulnerability. Continence might be more difficult for men, in a general sense, than for women, simply because men are not routinely subjected to monthly flows or to childbirth. What makes a man think of himself as masculine? As not a man, or half a man? These are social constructs, but they are rooted in physiology. The myth of male power has a great deal to do with the idea of containment.

Semen and urine share the same vessel, and that vessel isn't supposed to leak. In Philip Roth's novel *Exit Ghost,* Nathan Zuckerman, in the period following his prostatectomy, suffers both from incontinence and erectile dysfunction, changes so devastating that this fictional novelist drops out of the literary scene for a long time, holing himself up in a country house, daring only to swim in his own pond for fear of spontaneous urination while swimming laps at the college pool. He sends away for special leakproof pants ("bloomers," he calls them, designed to fit under swim trunks), but even those don't give him the confidence he needs.

Before treatment, Dean made a "deal" with God for continence. He got what he asked for—with modifications. He is continent now, but urinary function still needs the governing influences of Flomax, Pyridium, and Sanctura—three drugs that, working together, support predictable and manageable urination. Five percent of all men who choose brachytherapy will end up suffering, as Dean appears to, from "long-term persistent urinary dysfunction." Additionally, for brachytherapy patients like Dean who have enlarged prostates, the likelihood of such urinary dysfunction is much greater than it is for men with smaller glands. He is pleased that the medicines help him live in the world of continence as a normal citizen. Something else seems to have helped him regain control: about a year post-

WHAT WE KNOW NOW

Complementary medical approaches such as acupuncture, special diets, meditation, nutritional supplements, and support groups are all worth exploring; some health plans cover complementary medicine, and progressive hospitals may offer special clinics or consultations.

treatment, he had a series of acupuncture treatments, after which he was able to give up his continence pads.

Before that blessed return to almost-normal, traveling with pads had been hard for him to get used to. Without these aids, embarrassment can be overwhelming, as on a particular business flight into D.C. about a year and a half after 9/11, when passengers were forbidden to leave their seats during "lockdown." The pads were in his carry-on, he was strapped down, and the lavatory was off-limits.

Recently I have come to understand the meaning of "stress incontinence" myself. Six years after Dean's treatments began, I have to work at Kegel exercises, too, to defend against a surprise attack of convulsive laughter or a sneeze. These days, Dean is more practiced in this category than I am, a graduate of the school of urinary surprise.

What are the odds of getting continence back? Here are some recent numbers related to the main treatment approaches, all of which are described in Appendix A and the Glossary:

- *External beam radiation/TomoTherapy:* 10 to 15 percent chance of bladder and/or rectal irritation, and the long-term possibility of "persistent urinary dysfunction."
- *Prostatectomy:* 5 percent chance of permanent incontinence and 30 percent chance of stress urinary incontinence (in other words, involuntary actions such as sneezing or laughing may induce flow). Patients older than, say, sixty-seven are more

likely to suffer permanent incontinence after surgical removal of the prostate.

- *Brachytherapy:* Possibility of urinary urgency or urinary retention. A man treated with brachytherapy may be fine for a while, then suffer incontinence after a year or more. (Prostatectomy patients may find the opposite is true.) Five percent suffer long-term persistent urinary dysfunction.

Beyond the odds, here's how to stack the deck in favor of continence :

- *Pads or continence pants.* Use them, at least in the first few weeks or months, with no shame.
- *Kegel exercises.* These strengthen and increase the endurance of the pelvic floor muscles; they involve stopping, then restarting urinary flow while in progress, gradually increasing the time you hold the muscles tense. (See details in the Glossary.) The patient should, of course, consult with his urologist about when these simple exercises should begin.
- *Drugs to help regulate urination.* Flomax (and other alpha blockers) works by relaxing the bladder; Detrol and Sanctura (and other anti-cholinergics) decrease urinary spasms and frequency; and analgesics such as Pyridium relieve the burning sensation sometimes associated with post-treatment urination. These are very safe as drugs go, with long track records, and each aids a particular aspect of urination.
- Contrary to what would seem logical, *drink plenty of water.* Limit tea, coffee, alcohol, and spicy foods.
- *The "sling."* Installed surgically as an aid to continence for men who have lost urethral sphincter function and for men whose pelvic floor muscles have weakened. This is one of a few relevant minor surgeries, to be discussed with a urologist.
- *Collagen injections to strengthen bladder control.* In a study

published in September 2005 in *The Journal of Urology*, 322 men who were partially incontinent due to treatment for either prostate cancer or an enlarged prostate received a series of collagen injections into the "neck" of the bladder. After three years of follow-up, researchers found that men who had had their prostates removed and received the collagen injections had lowered their use of pads, and 17 percent of the overall population of men had achieved complete control over their bladders.

- *Acupuncture and/or biofeedback.* Acupuncture worked for Dean. Biofeedback, which utilizes electrical stimulation, has been helpful for some men. Don't be afraid to try these complementary techniques. They are painless, widely available, and covered by many medical plans.
- *Yoga and other forms of meditation.* Yogis demonstrate control over "involuntary" functions (such as blood pressure) when these functions were considered by Western medicine to be beyond the reaches of the human mind. (A recent visit to *Yoga Journal* on the Internet yielded a suggested exercise: see www.yogajournal.com/practice/1221.)

But incontinence is only half the struggle.

E.D. (IMPOTENCE)

We are the only species capable of fully realizing our own eroticism, something we have come to feel we ought to have access to anytime we please. Because women are regularly (not periodically) fertile, and because we humans are conscious of what we do, it is possible to focus purely on the pleasure our bodies offer and to forget that procreation was nature's original intent. The act of making love is complex, and it isn't granted to most of us in its natural spontaneous form for a lifetime, although we may think of it as artless, effortless, and endlessly available.

Given the heavy lifting involved, it's not surprising that a whole list of things can defeat a well-intended penis: performance anxiety, stress, fear, guilt, depression, pain, alcohol, a cold shower, sleep deprivation, boredom, nausea, plain old age, and a host of physiological conditions and treatment protocols, prostate cancer among them.

IN DEAN'S WORDS

I said to God, "Okay, here's the deal: leave me my dignity." I thought it was more important for a man in his fifties to keep his dignity—which meant, at the time, total continence—than to keep so-called potency. Then, about two weeks or so after the seeds were implanted and all that swelling went down, I thought I'd try to see if an erection might still happen. Things had ground to a halt sexually months before because of the hormones. Of course, nothing happened. I remained on hormone blockade.

After going to the new doctor, who agreed I should go off the hormone blockade, I gleefully flushed what was left of the pills down the toilet. Another few weeks followed before I ardently began to try once again to get an erection, but nothing happened.

I had won the bargain I made with God, but I guess I really never thought it would come to pass! I was surprised at how angry I was.

Then too, the penis is haunted by its emblematic cousin, the phallus: the rod of Aaron, the bolt of Zeus, the sword in the stone, a cigar (except, according to Freud, when that object is simply itself). But a penis isn't mythical, and for its owner it can be a terrible liability. It can express itself at the wrong times and fail when he needs it most.

In my dictionary, *potency* leads back to *potentatus*, Latin for "dominion." But what has erectile function got to do with any man's actual power, his robustness? Nothing, of course. Still, many men have a hard time seeing themselves as men without full erectile function, thanks to a youth-obsessed culture. Supposed to flourish until death, natural erectile ability often doesn't, which is quite normal. By age forty-five, most men have experienced at least some erectile dysfunction. Complete E.D. occurs for about 5 percent of men aged forty, 15 percent at seventy, and 50 to 70 percent between the ages of seventy and seventy-eight. So here's my question: But for describing jailed dictators, why do we need the word *impotent* at all? Language is powerful and labels are damaging; they can become prophetic.

I angrily resented Dean's bargain when I learned about it, some three or four years ago. It has been six long years, and only recently (largely on account of this book's genesis) have Dean and I begun to talk about what happened back then, about what we said, what we didn't say, what we did, and what we didn't do. For a long time I wondered if he had thought so little of our lovemaking that he would trade it for what I then thought of as the "convenience" of continence; but that is a feminine partner's perspective. After reading the testimonies of living prostate cancer survivors in Internet ListServs and elsewhere, I've come to understand how important urinary control is to most men.

Incontinence is actually more about loss of power than erectile function ever was, and the two are sometimes conflated. Dean thought, "If I ask for cancer to go away and then I ask to get everything back besides, I could lose the whole show, including my life." So the magical thinking ran, Don't ask for too much. Each case is different. In Dean's case, I think anger—at cancer, at one more disability beyond visual impairment—combined with the mind-changing aspects of androgen suppression and a lack of medical counseling on how to get things going again to send his libido AWOL.

Getting Some Form of Erectile Function Back, One Way or Another

Men "enjoy the simple mechanical aspect of pleasure more than women," writes Deborah Blum in *Sex on the Brain*. Indeed, 85 percent of married men report that they masturbate, compared with 45 percent of married women (although it has to be taken into account that men may be more willing to report honestly in this regard than women are). Many men with E.D. go to great expense and trouble, adjusting the cc's of the Caverject they inject into their penises (painless, apparently, if you know what you're doing) or ordering the right pump or rings or going for surgery to get an implant. Other men say, sadly, "It was good while it lasted." I can't imagine how difficult it is to lose that spontaneity, and men who have lost it have a right to be angry—and sad. The question is: Will they get some aspects of this function back? It depends.

A man who chooses to define sexuality as completely spontaneous and entirely dependent on a firm erection is setting the post-treatment bar very high. If, on the other hand, he can (as Dean is beginning to do) take an ironic or mildly humorous look at himself, then he may make some progress. For someone who has just emerged from treatment, "practicing" at erotic stimulation as soon as the doctor recommends it (assuming the doctor is willing to talk openly about sexual function in the first place) will increase the odds. New studies have shown that early use of Viagra-like medications may bring erectile function back sooner and in a larger percentage of men. Overall, depending on which procedures he has undergone, what his sexual life was like before treatment, who his partner is, and whether he is willing to use aids, the man may find a middle ground. He may even get almost full function back eventually; it's been known to happen!

Dean and I didn't do any of these things. He was too angry and proud, and I was too passive. Six years later, we're dealing with what we (and the first urologist) simply ignored. That doctor was reticent when it came to discussing post-treatment quality of life, let alone sexuality. And Dean felt humiliated, desexed, and silenced in the doctor's office. And because I had been shut out of office consultations with this urologist, I felt hesitant to approach Dean, afraid I would harm something. Urination felt to him like needles—a pain that sometimes lasted half an hour—so I was afraid to initiate anything. He always seemed so unapproachable, so touchy, twitchy, and "on fire."

After the radiation-engendered urinary fire more or less subsided—almost a year after treatment—we began to put our life back together; but the very definition of intimacy seemed to be up for grabs. We had been sleeping apart at his request, because he was constantly on the move, running down the hallway or writhing from muscle spasms. When we began occasionally sleeping together, we were confused, angry, and, frankly, out of practice! But the biggest wet blanket of all was that hormone ablation seemed, for Dean, to have completely erased his desire.

IN DEAN'S WORDS

Erectile dysfunction, what the hormones did or didn't do, the inability to feel sexy . . . what am I to do with all this? As far as the medical establishment is concerned, first you have the meds—Viagra, Cialis, and the like (these I can't hazard for fear of losing what vision I have)—then there are the toys, the injections, pumps, and implants, and even erotica you can buy from the Net. But what about desire?

Despite the bad beginning and the less-than-ideal treatment plan, over the years we have recovered some of what was lost by constantly working at redefining *intimacy*. Massage, listening to music while lying body to body on the sofa: these we have.

133

Once, about a year and a half ago, he passed me in the hallway. At that time I was in the throes of shingles, a wretched condition, an adult form of chicken pox, that affects the nerve endings on one side of the body. Since my right shoulder and chest could not tolerate even the touch of my hair, I was going about the house that month dressed in a kind of toga that left my right breast exposed. He glanced at me, then whispered, "I just had half a hubba!" We ran to the bedroom, but the impulse—both the desire and the erectile response—had melted like ice in July.

We try to build on that and other moments. Viagra and equivalent drugs are off-limits for Dean on account of his macular degeneration. Meanwhile, we hear varying stories about their success or failure with various men. They open blood vessels, a good thing; but they have nothing to do with desire. Dean has a horror of needles, so no penile injections for him. A penile implant? He may be ready to consider that sooner rather than later; but it is an uphill battle as long as libido is still the missing guest at our party. Are these the lingering effects of hormone suppression? Libido can, it seems, be permanently damaged, but it remains to be seen how much of that effect is organic and how much a psychological by-product. Hormone blockade has been linked in several studies to poor quality of life, regardless of what other treatment may or may not have been used.

A few months ago, I sat down with Dean on a Saturday morning. A thought had entered my mind, and I wanted to share it with him: "We could either make our physical life together a referendum on your feelings of inadequacy, or we could redefine our marriage in the physical sense as two people with a problem. We are side by side. Why is it necessary to go 360 degrees around the circle, when we could step next door?"

Why did it take me almost six years to utter that sentence?

We have the desire to have . . . desire. I recently downloaded a description of Tantric sex. Some post-PCa treatment couples have

IN DEAN'S WORDS

Why we had to come full circle about closeness instead of just stepping next door . . . well, I don't know. I think it's as much about the marriage as it is about the disease. How many marriages, by the time they are thirty or thirty-five years old, have their own built-in physical problems, a kind of sameness? Like so many marriages, ours might have been nearing that point, and then the fragile consideration of that problem was crushed by hormones, by cancer, by radiation. Considering the confluence of those things, we're fortunate to have come full circle. The ability to talk, to still be interested in each other, to still be viably concerned about my E.D. I don't care how long it took us to get here.

found a new intimacy by using some of these ancient exercises. Rumors of aphrodisiacs drift about on the Internet, some with great names like horny goat weed and Korean red ginseng. L-arginine, which, anecdotally, seems promising as regards erectile function, may be worth a try. We are currently considering yohimbine, a natural substance derived from the bark of an African tree and the predecessor, apparently, to Viagra. Our research is only just beginning, and each substance we decide to investigate has to be okayed by Dean's retinologist. And so we continue.

QUALITY OF LIFE

It is a gift that Dean has survived. But then you both begin to notice what's missing. Incontinence or E.D. or both remain for many men long after treatment. Lying, as it does, at a sensitive crossroads in the male body, the prostate cannot be treated or removed without disturbing urinary and erectile functions, whether short term or long

IN DEAN'S WORDS

I remember a spice store below Eighth Street when I was in my early twenties, and the moment you walked in, you knew this wasn't just about cooking. Who knew what was for sale there in the back if you knew what to say? Aphrodisiacs? "Who the hell needs that?" I wondered back then, and anyhow, what would it do to you? I had so much energy and sexual vigor. At that age, just the thought of an aphrodisiac was scary. Now, I yearn for one of them to be real.

term, with possible implications for the bowel as well. Hormone ablation may cause a drop in libido, rise in weight, and onset of lethargy and depression. Various medical conditions may also ensue: anemia, diabetes, coronary disease, osteoporosis, high blood pressure, even possible cognitive decline. This grim list largely describes patients who have stayed on the hormone ablation treatments for longer than six months. Treatment and post-treatment effects may be subtle or not-so-subtle and differ for every individual. In other words, choose what you will—aside from "watchful waiting," there will be changes in his body. So your life and your relationship will change, too; how could they not?

That said, here are some suggestions for working to increase erectile function:

- *Practice makes better,* if not perfect—and whatever you do, do it *with no shame.*
- *A sense of humor helps,* with a tinge of irony if you can manage it.
- *Viagra, Cialis, and similar drugs* work only where libido is still present.
- *So-called aphrodisiacs.* Ask your doctor about substances such as yohimbine, horny goat weed, and Korean red gin-

seng, but don't expect official medical encouragement. If you're told it's safe for you, then try it. You never know.

- *Caverject (alprostadil) and similar injectable drugs.* Many men swear by this method, and apparently if you know what you're doing, it isn't painful. A man injects himself with a "local" version of what Viagra and Cialis deliver. Priapism (an erection that refuses to leave) is sometimes a liability. A lot depends on the fine-tuning of the dose (see Michael Korda's description of his own priapism experience in his memoir of prostate cancer, *Man to Man*).

- *Vacuum erection devices.* These are mechanical pumps that draw blood into the penis; a constriction band placed at the base of the penis sustains the erection and may be kept in place safely for half an hour.

- *Penile implant.* Some men undergo an operation: the installation of a penile prosthesis that they can make erect at will. Many good accounts of penile implants come over the Internet; do your own research.

- *Think about sensuality in a relaxed ("nonphallocentric") context.* Why does the penis have to be the star of the show? Why does the man have to be the prime mover?

- *Talk* about what has happened between the two of you. Express everything, but personalize nothing (easier said than done).

- *Be willing to let go of the idea of total spontaneity.* Planning has to enter the picture. This is actually true for most people in or beyond middle age, but especially for prostate cancer survivors. This may be the hardest single aspect of reclaiming sexual intimacy.

Identity—male, that is—gives incontinence and "impotence" almost equal weight. Before prostate cancer entered our lives, I never gave a thought to either, but if asked, I would have said that incontinence is merely an inconvenience, an embarrassment best

---

WHAT WE KNOW NOW

I wish someone (the urologist?) had told us back then how important it is to try right away to get erectile function back. The longer you wait, the more challenging the process is.

---

managed with pads and other aids, whereas erectile dysfunction threatens identity. Now I know how important they both are. The ability to govern bodily fluids of any kind is, for most men (Dean included), a kind of power, and the loss of either kind of governance leaves a man vulnerable in ways that may call into question who he is. So it has been with Dean, and many of his doctors (all men) have seemed, over time, reticent to speak frankly or humanly about either of these losses.

THE CONTROVERSY SURROUNDING TESTOSTERONE REPLACEMENT

Andropause (as discussed in chapter 6) is not only a popular topic these days; it has fueled a medical industry. In "Hormones for Men: Is Male Menopause a Question of Medicine or of Marketing?" (*The New Yorker*, July 29, 2002), Jerome Groopman expresses considerable doubts about whether there is such a definable stage of development for men. What's not in doubt is that male menopause is a marketing concept that has facilitated the promotion of testosterone patches—hormone replacement therapy—to men unafflicted with prostate cancer who may have decreased libido, lack of energy, lost height, less strong erections, depression, a deterioration in ability to play sports, or a deterioration in work performance. Some of these men perceive themselves to be in, or near, andropause, assuming that state actually exists.

How muddy these waters truly are. Many men drift gradually into a low-energy state during their fifties and sixties, even without the dampening effects of prostate cancer treatments. The possible existence of "male menopause" and the recent marketing of testosterone replacement for the general population can make men who have already undergone treatment for prostate cancer feel even more confused or angry.

Some "feel-good" doctors peddle testosterone—for both men and women—as a panacea to cure many ills, in addition to staving off "andropause." How tempting it must be to go for testosterone patches if you've had androgen ablation, radiation, or other libidinally depleting treatments; but testosterone is a hazard for this population.

There are men who have, despite the warnings of urologists, put on testosterone patches after cancer treatments to revive their youthful selves. General medical wisdom to date holds that it is, sadly, imprudent to risk waking up the "sleeping giant" of cancer this way.

CHAPTER ELEVEN

THE BODY IN BED:

What Do You Miss? What Do You Need?

LIKE WATER on an old roof, cancer (if patient and partner survive) finds all the cracks and weak spots. Four and a half years after diagnosis, why has it taken us so long to speak to each other about what happened?

Sometimes on Sunday nights, we fight. He comes off a working weekend exhausted, only wanting to crawl into bed. That's reasonable, but he would usually rather crawl in there alone. And I never understand. I always take it as rejection, the most personal kind. That's because we aren't lovers anymore. We were losing that connection when the treatment protocols began, and now what's left?

Wouldn't a man who's been away all weekend want a warm body in the bed next to him? An insomniac wouldn't, especially if the body next to him snores. We used to cuddle with fierce intimacy every night, and that cuddling made all the difference to me. Without it, I am inconsolably lonely. Meanwhile, alone in his bed these days, he gets at least some of the sleep he needs.

Now here's the part that makes me crazy, one of the roof cracks cancer has found: I fear sometimes that he never really wanted me, my body, that is. I know how much he loves my mind. Perhaps he was always more interested in friendship, conversation, good meals, movies, music. Companionship. Often it's the wife who's "relieved" when sex is over. Are we the reverse couple? So I fear.

This journal entry seems to have drifted back from a lost decade, but I wrote it only last year.

MOVE BEYOND THE IDEA OF PERFORMANCE

That is a command; I take it as such, at any rate, a message from the unconscious. Moving beyond the idea of (sexual) performance is just what we have been trying to do. Recently, we've taken a few important steps. When I suggested to Dean that our physical life together had become a "referendum on his feelings of inadequacy," I meant it; and I was pleased that he seemed to find this a fascinating idea. He's happy to surrender his lead role in the recent "reclaiming sexual intimacy" drama. And anyway, performance is boring! Not to mention superficial.

Take, for example, performance-enhancing drugs, the secret vice of so many baseball players and Olympic professionals. How are these any different from Viagra or Cialis? After all, both are physical and rely on a physiological ideal. The (slight) difference, it seems to me, is that one "performance" is private and the other public. But wait. Why do we have to fight off this phony approach to sex? Well, consider that our culture seems almost to encourage sex as a competitive sport; a lot of bragging seems to surround the subject, and any adult who hasn't had sex in a few months, let alone a whole year, is considered abnormal. Now think how easy it is for a man recovering from any of several prostate cancer treatments to feel defeated, whether by a dampened libido or by an unwilling penis. I have read so many chronicles of post–prostate cancer marriages like ours: struggling, dissolving, not dissolving, coming together heroically, falling apart, or growing somehow in spite of what is lost, growing, as Eve's did (from chapter 1), out of the very pit and pith of cancer itself (remember, she began dating her husband right after his diagnosis). There are some prostate cancer stories that, in time, resolve themselves; all of them seem to ditch the notion of male sexual "performance," either eventually or right away.

That throws the woman into the lead role, or at least into the role of catalyst. Raised as I was in the good old bad old days of strong man/submissive woman, I have always found doing the seducing a little like defying gravity. It's scary, especially now that I am beyond middle age; and post-treatment (after testosterone was nearly eliminated), it's harder than ever to be the seducer. It's so easy to lose all grace in this role, because something essential is entirely missing, which must be reinvented—no, *reimagined.*

IN DEAN'S WORDS

What do I miss? I'm a great reader of junk, what I call high-class trash—on tape, of course. Mysteries and grown boys' adventures. I'm reading a mystery now where the hero gets himself put into jail to find out what's going on . . . because the bad guy's in jail. The protagonist is in there for about a week, he's beaten up, but finally he uncovers the plot, and he goes home to have his first night back together with his girlfriend. Well, his lawyer, who has given them his house so they can have the first night back together, observes, "First-night-back-together sex is even better than make-up sex." I have no idea what it's like to come out of jail, but I do remember "make-up sex," and I miss it. First the disagreement, then the sex, and finally the cuddling. The misunderstanding, then: "Let's just make love."

I find it sometimes incomprehensible to look back on me, on Dean as a twenty-three-year-old who, just as naturally as nowadays I shower or let the dogs out for a run, would roll over and make love to Vicki.

Even with the possibility of aphrodisiacs, injections, an implant, whatever—it's spontanaeity I miss . . . the naturalness of my life. But how much of that might have happened gradually, anyway? I have never been sixty-two before. I was fifty-six when I was diagnosed. But I do know that after Lupron and Casodex and radiation, I'm different. I'll add that difference to a list of other things I lost long ago. For example, I miss not being able to run fast and pick the ball off the turf and roll with it against my chest for a completed pass. Football: that's something I've missed for a lot longer.

Right now, most of all, I miss the spontanaeity of sex, which was taken from me suddenly.

What do I miss? The spontaneity that always started our love-making was, I think, already beginning to erode when cancer came along. Then the treatments killed spontaneous desire for Dean and left me fumbling in the dark.

I miss being desired—that is a woman's true power. I treasure the moment over a year ago when he saw me in my "toga" and had "half a hubba." To me, that proves that his libido is still in there, like the prince in a fairy tale, asleep for a hundred years in a castle, just enchanted. What are the words to break the spell?

I miss being sexy in a general sense. That may be like Dean's catching the football pass, because you're a young woman walking down the street, you get all this attention—you're afraid of it or, back when feminism was making us see things differently, you get angry at the guys in hard hats and the wolf whistles. Wow, do I miss those insults now! I miss the feeling of being in danger crossing Central Park in a miniskirt. Not being noticed is the female equivalent of what they call *impotence*—that word fits here, because your power as a (hetero) woman when it comes to sex is in *his* physical response.

What I don't have anymore is the knowledge that somebody else lying right next to me feels something like what I'm feeling. If he felt that way but just couldn't act on it, even if there was no real remedy for not being able to act, then I'd feel less lonely. To me, the loss of erectile function is a very big inconvenience, but libido's absence is devastating.

I used to say that I miss cuddling, but that has blessedly returned. Well, mostly returned, because as long as his insomnia and my snoring exist as incompatible systems, and as long as the work world beckons five days a week, we cuddle on schedule, usually on the weekends.

IN DEAN'S WORDS

What do I need? I need . . . the confidence to allow her to make moves without fear of failure. I miss, I need . . . calmness. Once, two or three years ago when I went for a blood test, my urologist said, "What's the occasion?" I was in a dark suit, white shirt, formal tie. "Nothing," I replied; "just a client meeting." "Client meeting?" he says. "You mean, you've been working all this time?" I guess he thought I was retired.

Because I worked the whole time cancer was going on in post-9/11 New York, keeping my business going in a recession, I miss the calmness that I think retirement may bring in conjunction with this disease. How different this disease must be for an older population. Would I have had the time and energy to deal more squarely with cancer if I hadn't been constantly pulled toward work?

What do I need? I wrote this book to keep from going crazy, and to get Dean's attention. I need my husband back, perhaps not *exactly* as he was when he was snatched from me so suddenly. But when it comes to sex and sensuality, I need him to be willing to try for less than perfection. He's been fine, quite workmanlike, when it comes to issues of continence; he knows which medicines he has to take, and he practices strengthening his pelvic floor muscles; he accepts who he is in that arena.

When it comes to physical intimacy, I know I have to take the initiative; but it's really hard to be the only person with a libido! It's lonely; you feel like a drag on the other person, and for someone who was raised to be pretty conventionally "feminine," it's a difficult role. I find it really easy to talk myself out of trying, because being rejected hurts so much.

I am so pleased that he wants, finally, to try again, however unspontaneous the result might end up being. I think he is beginning to miss desire and wants to find a way to reconstruct it or to create something new in its place. The final healing, I think, is in making the old new.

"HOW DID CANCER CHANGE YOUR LIVES IN PUBLIC AND IN PRIVATE?": VOICES OF WIVES AND PARTNERS

LIZ

The hardest thing for me personally has been the feeling that I can't or shouldn't discuss his impotence with anyone. I have referred to it vaguely with my sister and feel as if I am betraying him. I guess I have suppressed my sadness even from myself for a long time. I don't want to discuss my feelings with him because I don't want to make him feel sadder. I don't want him to feel like he's a failure, because he isn't. Medically, he is a success: he is cured. I can't and won't open up to my girlfriends about this, because that would be betraying him. Talking about mild incontinence occasionally with others is almost but not quite in the same category. My personal isolation is the biggest problem for me. I know there is help out there, but I don't think I can reach out for it, at least not yet.

ANGIE

Sickness can actually improve a relationship; you wouldn't choose it, but Clark is more in touch with what some might call his "feminine" side since his cancer. He would talk about mortality openly after diagnosis. He thought a lot more than I did about his impotence, and he talked about it. We'd already been to couples therapy . . . my need for intimacy, you see, was always different than his, so we had had to go. After cancer? His libido was not affected; E.D., yes, to a point—but he can take Viagra and it's fine. Because of cancer, he could allow someone to take care of him. That was a good, close time.

EVE

Well, Harry was given a book of reflections—one for every day of the year—and it's interesting how he has come to use it. He's really taken a shine to this beautiful book; it lies open on the table by the window, and every morning he flips through it randomly and reads whatever his finger falls on. We either ruminate on it and take it to heart or laugh out loud, either one or the other. What I love about him is that there is a kind of peace and built-in calm. I didn't know him before cancer, because we met right after diagnosis, but I think that somehow this calm, this taking each day as it comes, probably has something to do with what he went through. Sometimes I even think he is naive, then I think, well, maybe I'm naive too. I keep wondering why he reacts so much to the PSA tests every six months! Then I think there's a part of me that really doesn't know what he is going through.

ELIZABETH

You might say that our stars collided: his prostate cancer and my breast cancer. He was seventy-six and I was sixty-eight. We went through radiation together; there really was no "well partner" around the house to worry about the "sick partner." We were both facing very common diseases for our ages (every other man in our retirement village has had a bout of prostate cancer, and so many women I know have had breast cancer). His PSA was at 9 and then rose quickly, so the doctor did a biopsy. He told Michael, "You're positive for prostate cancer," then added, calmly, "but you'll die of something else, not this." He assured us, "if it recurs, we'll use hormones." Michael's sex life had been inactive for several years, so there wasn't much of a change in that sense, but the urinary problems were a trial for him. It does change your lives, though, even at our age—in the sense that it reminds you how close you are to death. Past seventy, it's simply a different disease.

CHAPTER TWELVE

THE ART OF DAILY SURVIVAL:
Everything Old Is New Again

THE PROSTATE GLAND plays a vital supporting role in the drama of babymaking. Because the gland often doesn't cause its owner noticeable difficulties—that is, become enlarged or cancerous—until late in life, when the drama of fertility is likely to have been concluded, it is possible for a man to go forever without knowing what his prostate is or does. I certainly didn't know.

I thought, mistakenly, that the prostate's role somehow had to do with the production of sperm. I've since learned that the prostate simply *nourishes* the sperm. In other words, it isn't the star of the procreative play, but perhaps the stagehand. In the standard medical definition: "The primary function of the prostate gland is to produce semen. Semen consists of proteins and other chemicals that *nourish* [my italics] the sperm and are critical to male fertility. The portion of the semen made in the prostate helps preserve and transport the sperm that are formed in the testicles and stored in the adjacent epididymis. Without the prostate, reproduction through sexual intercourse would be impossible."

At first, the word *nourish* seemed odd to me in this context, like an astrologer at a party of nuclear physicists. How exactly does a gland nourish? But then I looked it up in my trusty *Webster's*. Defi-

148

nition #1 fits the prostate's role perfectly: "To sustain with food or nutriment, to supply with what is necessary for life, health, and growth." So the prostate supplies what is necessary for fertility health.

But if the prostate's role is largely reproductive (not somehow magically involved with "manhood" or the mechanics of erection), then preserving it if your reproductive years are over seems foolish. How many men have made ignorant treatment choices based on a poor understanding of what their prostate actually does?

HEALING BEYOND THE CURE

So I ask myself, "What am I nourishing, writing this book?" It is a cautionary tale, a "don't do what we did" kind of story. The negatives are obvious and provocative. But on the positive side, this book is an odd kind of valentine to my husband, who wanted to turn his back on the aftermath of cancer and treatment, and the way these things had changed our daily life together, and walk away. It is natural to want to walk away after cancer, but in this case it wasn't going to work, because one person had cancer but two people suffered, and lots of things were going unsaid.

"Because I—we—are writing this book, our life has changed," I tell myself sometimes, and I list all the things that wouldn't be happening if I hadn't started writing what eventually became the first chapter.

We are redefining intimacy—through music, through massage, through plain old touching. There are aphrodisiacs and "toys" and so much stuff we have only, finally, begun to embark on, things we know about largely because this book made me find out about them.

We have a community: we are members of Man to Man, and every month we meet the newly diagnosed who may be helped by our story. We met Elaine and Peter Albert through our mutual veterinarian, but our deep relationship with them is nourished—to borrow from that lively description of the prostate's role—by the monthly meetings of Man to Man we all attend, and by the support group What About Me?, which Elaine started with my help. These are all gifts that Dean's cancer inadvertently bestowed: an abiding friendship and a group of people who wouldn't be meeting if there had been no cancer to begin with.

The inadvertence of these gifts is what allows me to be grateful to cancer for them. I happen to be looking right now at Long Island Sound. At high tide or during a storm, the sea finds a particular rock crevice. It may or may not leave that crevice intact, but it does leave occasional prizes. Like the sea with its smoothed bits of glass, cancer leaves random gifts: a friend, a lesson, even a book. It's not the cancer that you're grateful for, of course, but its gifts are worth acknowledging. And then, if cancer leaves you each grateful for the next breath you take, that may be the only gift equal in weight to such a crisis.

I miss our old life, wouldn't be human if I didn't. I recently reread chapter 1, the month of not-knowing, and wanted to linger there and not read on, to stay forever in the *before* that precedes the *after* of treatment.

But here we are in the *after*. For the rest of his life, Dean will go for a blood test every six months and, we hope, breathe easier afterward; so it goes for any cancer patient post-treatment. Each negative result is a blessing. "Could last a full lifetime, if we're lucky," he pointed out once, which is to say: *you live until you die.* This book has healed us, possibly even saved our marriage. In the conversations it has engendered, the friends we've met, and the communities we've joined, it has brought us closer. So then, cancer, which once came between us like a knife, has lost the fight.

THESE DAYS

We sleep together much of the time now; cuddling is sweet and tender. Humor, sharpened by a new sense of irony, is more delicious than ever. Dean looks so young, a man of sixty-two who still has a

IN DEAN'S WORDS

I've been in one or another kind of show business venture my entire life. Back when we were in our twenties, we took the lease on a movie palace, a grand old theater down the block from where we still live in Staten Island. I foresaw a great entertainment space, including children's theater, rock concerts, film, jazz—but I'd failed to notice that we lived in a community that didn't really want what we had to offer. We went bankrupt in a year, failed completely, miserably.

I got a job. The quickest way to the ferry and then to the city was down Hyatt Street, beneath the blank marquee of the vacant theater we had gone broke trying to run. To avoid walking past the theater, I would have had to go at least four blocks and ten minutes out of my way. Sometimes if the day hadn't been particularly fruitful, I took the long way home.

To walk past the scene of my greatest failure almost every single day was ultimately good for me. This book has been much the same: it has been the "marquee" of the last few years of my life. It's our story, the years that made me who I am, my decisions, both good and bad. We've met some fine people along the way and a few good doctors. Some mediocre ones, too.

I should have reached out to Vicki sooner.

You out there, whether diagnosed or soon to be treated, cancer survivor or spouse, if you don't have a mate, find a friend, find anybody to talk to. Find a group, if you can. Don't get stuck in your own anger or self-pity. Get more than one opinion and try to understand what prostate cancer is, instead of just reacting. Look deep inside yourself. Whether or not I made the best choice, it worked out for me: I'm healthy now, wiser than I was before. Be well in your journey and get well. Talk to people. Whatever you do, just don't do it alone.

full head of blond hair. People routinely mistake him for a man ten years younger. He has recovered most of his original energy, and his digestion has improved (he astonished me the other day by suggesting we go for Indian food!), reminding me how important the small stuff truly is.

Now we stand together on the cusp of what we hope is another thirty years. If this is extreme optimism, why not? As his dad, raised in the Great Depression, used to say about optimism, "After all, it doesn't cost anything." Beyond any cost, I am attracted to the notion of the mind and body as a continuum; and so, isn't it important to imagine yourself as healthy and as living a long life?

Many aren't as lucky as we have been. There are those whose diagnoses came too late. Many men got the disease before early diagnosis was possible, when treatments weren't as sophisticated as they are today. Three of the seventeen men in Dean's original treatment group died in the treatment year. It's all so complex, and technology is a racehorse. I fully expect to wake some morning to the news that all the current treatments, with their damaging side effects, have been rendered obsolete by some new streamlined procedure. Some are already in the works. A rumored vaccine? Who knows?

All cancers may someday be "chronic" maladies, to be treated as such. Will doctors in this not-so-distant future be better able to translate the complexities of the new technology to their patients? Will official health care begin to recognize the changes—emotional and physical—wives and husbands must undergo as a result of any of the various protocols that make up prostate cancer treatment?

A persistent notion (reinforced by the egos of some doctors and researchers) that there is one true holy grail of prostate cancer treatment—combined with the complexities of science, the intricacies of the male body, and basic human fear—make treatments for this disease seem like a labyrinth with no real exit.

While we're waiting for the ultimate cure, where is the mandated counseling for any man and partner preparing to undergo the chemical castration hell of hormone ablation? Where is the hefty manual comparing all current treatment strategies dispassionately, with allowances for such things as age, prostate size, even lifestyle? Where is the honest list of unpleasant side effects? The current Medicaid director of Nebraska recently announced that the state intends to drop funding for Viagra and penile implants—in short, funding for aids to erectile dysfunction—because "sex is not medically necessary." The fact that a substantial percentage of men with E.D. have it as a result of prostate cancer left her unfazed. Not necessary?

Without sexual identity, who are we?

Science has got some things so very right; now for the human part, where we learn the art of daily survival.

A Crash Course in
Current Treatment Options

Here I have condensed what you might find in a number of books, articles, and Web sites on prostate cancer treatment. It is not intended as a substitute for medical advice from a qualified physician.

PROSTATECTOMY

This is the most established treatment method, involving the surgical removal of the prostate gland. Ask your urologist for an in-depth explanation of the major variations. They include: retropubic, perineal, laparoscopic, robotic, and pelvioscopic. These procedures differ either in actual surgical approach (*retropubic*, for example, means "behind the pubic bone") or tool use, as in robotic (when the surgeon operates utilizing a robot). Again, ask your urologist for the subtle—and strategic—differences between them. Because the prostate contains certain nerve bundles that are crucial to erectile function, a "nerve-sparing" radical prostatectomy (laparoscopic, robotic, or pelvioscopic) is usually recommended wherever possible *if* the PSA is 10 or higher and Gleason grade is 6 or lower.

Patients preparing for prostatectomy may be advised to give blood in advance, and should expect to stay in the hospital several days. With its four-to-six-week recovery period (including seven to ten days of catheterization), prostatectomy is major surgery. All prostatectomies should result in a PSA at undetectable levels, assuming no cancer cells have been left behind.

Possible side effects with retropubic (traditional) prostatectomy include: less than 5 percent incidence of permanent incontinence, 30 percent risk of stress urinary incontinence, and 50 percent incidence of E.D. Despite nerve-sparing techniques, there can be nerve or rectal injury. Although laparoscopic and robotic methods seem to allow faster recovery and a greater chance of returned normal function, long-term data are not yet available for these surgical techniques.

EXTERNAL BEAM RADIATION AND IMRT
(INTENSITY MODULATED RADIATION THERAPY)

IMRT is a refinement of the original external beam method, defined as radiation (some 7,500 rads) passing through skin tissue and focusing for maximal effect on its target: the prostate. In each of these methods, a beam of radiation is passed into the afflicted organ; IMRT and TomoTherapy, however, are more targeted approaches, so are less likely to damage surrounding organs and tissues. With either treatment, the patient makes visits five days a week for approximately eight to nine weeks, and receives his treatments while lying on a table.

Possible side effects of external beam treatments include fatigue, skin reaction in treated areas, and proctitis (rectal bleeding—a 30 percent chance). Rarely, there may be blood in the urine and, very rarely, frequent stools or abnormal bowel function. There is a 30 to 50 percent chance of E.D., 10 to 15 percent chance of bladder and/or rectal irritation, and the long-term possibility of persistent urinary dysfunction. PSA may not go to undetectable levels, as it should with surgery, but will reach its lowest value at five years, and should stay in this range if the treatment is successful.

PROTON BEAM THERAPY

Similar to external beam treatments, this approach substitutes proton beams for radiation, which, it is theorized, are more targeted than even the most targeted IMRT, "a type of radiation therapy that uses nuclear technology to precisely shoot fast-moving ions into tumors" (*U.S. News & World Report*, January 2008). As of this writing, randomized trials for this approach are yet to be done, making claims that the approach reduces complications hard to verify. The huge expense of outfitting a hospital for this approach has curtailed its widespread use to date. There are currently five places in the U.S. where it is operational, beginning with Loma Linda in California, where it originated in the early 1990s.

BRACHYTHERAPY

This treatment involves the implantation of radioactive pellets, or "seeds," throughout the prostate via needle punctures, an outpatient surgical procedure. A team of three—a radiation oncologist, a urologist, and a radiation dosimetrist—cooperate in the highly strategic placement of the seeds via long needles, utilizing sonographic and fluoroscopic monitoring. A computer determines the number and placement of seeds. In this approach, the radiation oncologist is the head strategist, the urologist acts as the surgeon, and the dosimetrist verbally instructs in seed placement.

Iodine-125, palladium-103, and, more recently, cesium are the seeds of choice. Cesium is the "new kid on the block," whereas iodine and palladium have longer track records. Iodine seeds are radioactive for up to six months, palladium seeds for only two. Because brachytherapy is a kind of "smart bomb"—irradiating only the prostate—it employs as many as 12,500 rads. The precise targeting and increased dose may be its greatest selling points. Combination therapies—brachytherapy with an external beam "boost," for a possible total of 14,500 rads—are also available for higher-risk patients with T2 tumors and Gleason grades of 7 or higher, or for very young patients who do not elect radical prostatectomy.

Brachytherapy is the treatment most often touted as minimally invasive: no hospitalization, no incisions, no transfusions. Even with the added rads of an external beam boost, however, men with high-grade cancers are more likely to fail—that is, to require (often less effective) salvage treatment later on. It is also, regardless of the grade of the cancer, difficult to seed a large prostate, which may require a course of hormone ablation to shrink the gland down to a suitable size for seed implantation. Possible side effects, in some cases permanent, include burning, urinary urgency, rectal irritation, bowel urgency (rare), pain during ejaculation, and urinary retention. Men receiving brachytherapy are counseled not to sit close to pregnant women or to hold babies during the time that their seeds are radioactive. The chance of E.D. runs anywhere from 25 to 60 percent. In the short term, with localized cancer (totally within the prostate capsule), this treatment appears to be curative.

CRYOSURGERY

With this treatment (also known as cryotherapy), the prostate is frozen to destroy the cancer cells. It's often used as a salvage method (on patients previously treated, for whom cancer has recurred). Possible treatment side effects beyond E.D. and incontinence include irritation of the rectal wall, irritation of the urethra, urethral scar formation, and urethrorectal fistula—an association between the rectum and the urethra that can lead to leakage and infections. Cryotherapy's effectiveness as an initial treatment strategy has not yet been well established; some sources list this approach, at least for initial treatment, as "experimental."

HORMONE ABLATION

Hormone therapy is a "palliative" treatment—that is, it's not, by itself, curative. Essentially, hormones are administered to halt testosterone production, thus killing around 90 percent of the cancer cells (the ones dependent on testosterone for growth). Variations include: orchiectomy (a surgical procedure that quickly drops testosterone to almost zero and is permanent), injection therapy (at intervals, usually monthly), or an anti-androgen (daily pill: Casodex, Nilandron, Eulexin), to stop adrenal testosterone production. Anti-androgen pills are often used in conjunction with injections, a combination that forms a "blockade" eliminating the production of testosterone by both the prostate and the adrenal gland. Hormone therapies or blockades are often used to assist radiation (especially with brachytherapy), as some prostates must be reduced in size before seed implantation.

Temporary side effects include hot flashes, lethargy, depression, weight gain, breast enlargement, E.D., and lack of libido (but E.D. and lack of libido may be permanent). Orchiectomy may involve infection, bleeding, or pain. Anti-androgens have various side effects, with possible implications for the liver, the heart, the bones (osteoporosis), and the lungs.

Dr. Martin Sanda, lead researcher of a recent quality-of-life study involving all major treatment protocols, told the *Wall Street Journal* that findings would "throw a splashful of cold water" on the use of hormone therapy in less severe cancers.

HIFU (HIGH-INTENSITY FOCUSED ULTRASOUND)

High-intensity focused ultrasound, which does not have approval in the United States to date, is similar to what happens when a magnifying glass collects heat from the sun. No radiation is used (it's computer-driven, as is brachytherapy); a probe that is sufficiently hot to melt the lipids in cells is inserted in the rectum during an outpatient procedure. This approach is apparently targeted (as is IMRT) and can avoid, its proponents claim, the urinary, sphincter, and neurovascular "bundles," the sensitive nerves that make erectile function possible.

Beyond Europe, where the treatment is in wide use, HIFU is also available in Canada and the Caribbean. Long-range statistics available from European studies are not officially recognized here. Some Americans choose to fly abroad for these treatments.

CHEMOTHERAPY

Often listed as palliative, chemotherapy is not, to date, a major treatment for prostate cancer, but is sometimes brought into play as a salvage method, when other treatments fail or when cancer has returned. The following chemotherapy drugs have been used to increase quality of life and slow advanced cancers: paclitaxel (Taxol), docetaxel (Taxotere), mitoxantrone (Novantrone), estramustine phosphate (Emcyt), etoposide (Vepsid), doxorubicin (Adriamycin), vinblastine (Velban), and carboplatinum.

MAJOR FACTORS AFFECTING
TREATMENT CHOICES

There is no "best" treatment—no "one size fits all," or even fits most. Prostate cancer treatment choice is, of course, entirely personal, and, as the public service announcement on my local jazz station reminds me daily, "prostate cancer is 90 percent curable if caught in time." But each case is different. Five factors conspire to complicate an already complicated decision-making process: PSA, Gleason grades, stage of the cancer, size of the prostate, and age and relative robustness (general medical status) of the patient. Here's a quick review of the first three: PSA, Gleason grade, and clinical staging.

PSA stands for prostate-specific antigen, a chemical produced naturally that shows up both in benign and malignant prostate tissue. Since PSA levels tend to be higher when cancer is present, it serves as a marker. A high PSA does not necessarily indicate the presence of cancer, but a gradually rising PSA is a reason for concern and scrutiny.

The *Gleason grade* is a widely used system for classifying the appearance of cancerous cells. The less they resemble normal cells, the more malignant the cancer. Every Gleason grade includes two numbers, from 1 to 5, for the two types of cancer cells, major and minor. These numbers are added together (3 + 3, or 4 + 3, for example). A Gleason of 7 or above is more critical; and the first number, representing major cells, is the more significant, as it represents the major pattern.

159

(Clinical) staging helps doctors determine whether the cancer is confined to the prostate and, if it is not, where and how much it has spread. This assessment is made by digital rectal exam and/or bone or CT scan. There are several staging systems, but the most common one bears the acronym TNM (T = size of tumor, N = node involvement, M = cancer metastasized outside the prostate and lymph nodes). Within the T category, you may see T1a, T2b, and so on. These further distinctions refer to where the cancer is located (in one or both lobes of the prostate) and whether or to what extent it has spread outside the prostate capsule. A T1a (found, incidentally, in less than 5 percent of the prostate tissue) is the least dangerous cancer, using this staging system. (See also *clinical staging* in the Glossary.)

As this is no textbook, I'll leave hair splitting to the experts. It is wise to discuss staging, PSA, and Gleason grading in detail with the urologist you and your partner have chosen.

Age of the patient and *prostate size* are the wild cards. Beyond sixty-five, it may be neither necessary nor prudent to undergo a radical prostatectomy (removal of the prostate). This may be true of some men slightly younger than sixty-five as well, if their health is fragile. With a four-to-six-week healing time, the possible need for two units of blood, catheterization, and a minimum two-day hospital stay, this is a serious—and delicate—operation. The prostate is at the equivalent of a three-way intersection: the bladder and bowel are its intimate neighbors. How close, for example, is the bladder wall to the rectum? As close, apparently, as wallpaper is to a wall. A man whose urinary function is entirely healthy going into the operation stands about a 20 percent chance of developing stress incontinence from weakened pelvic floor muscles; a much older man may suffer permanent and total incontinence. After prostatectomy, a healthy man still on the young side of his sixties should avoid lifting objects heavier than 20 pounds for as long as six weeks.

Beyond prudence, why is it not (in many cases) necessary to remove the cancerous prostates of men in their late sixties and beyond? This cancer is famously glacial in speed, and that speed gets even slower as the body ages. A man of seventy with PSA less than 4, Gleason 6, Stage T1c, may expect, if he does nothing at all, to die of some other malady. Men beyond their sixties often go for "active surveillance" (watchful waiting) or palliative care (hormone ablation by itself). Of the major treatments, there are always beam radiation and seeds. These may be the ideal treatments for men sixty-five to seventy-two or seventy-three. Some urologists call these "the radiation years."

Now drop the age clock back below sixty-five. All the major treatments have similar statistics for no recurrence at fifteen years. But at greater than fifteen years, only prostatectomy is statistically reliable in this regard. There is such a thing as "salvage prostatectomy," but it is difficult and risky: the possibilities for damaging the rectum are apparently considerable. Cryo methods, chemo, and hormone ablation are largely what remain for a radiation patient whose cancer has returned.

Prostate size is another factor. Dean underwent eight months of hormone ablation, which has radically affected his quality of life. Although this treatment kills approximately 90 percent of the testosterone-dependent cancer cells, that's not the whole story as to why he underwent hormone therapy. His prostate was enlarged to begin with (90.3 grams), too large for efficient seed implantation. The larger the prostate, the harder it is to successfully target the cancer with seeds and the more postoperative residual urinary problems may occur. Men in Dean's original support group with similar stats but smaller prostates merely got the seeds; so some libidos were left intact, and most are not troubled, as he still is, with persistent urinary difficulties.

Temporary or Permanent Side Effects
of Hormone Ablation

For an excellent text regarding hormone therapy and attendant side effects, please see Brad Guess, "Preventing and Treating the Side Effects of Testosterone Deprivation Therapy in Men with Prostate Cancer: A Guide for Patients and Physicians" (www.prostatecancer.org/education/andind/ Guess_TestosteroneSideEffects.html).

There are basically two types of medical hormone therapies: luteinizing hormone-releasing analogs, or LHRH (such as Lupron, Viadur, Eligard, and Zoladex), and oral anti-androgens (such as Eulexin, Nilandron, and Casodex). What follows is a list of possible side effects.

Bear in mind that hormone therapies may affect blood pressure or cholesterol and have implications for diabetes, incidence of stroke, heart health, and bone density—so a thorough workup before the treatment process begins is prudent. Duration of treatment is a serious topic for discussion.

• *Lethargy.* Testosterone is a prime mover, and its loss will be felt. Get moving, if you can—exercise!

• *Breast growth and/or loss of muscle tone.* These may be permanent, but you can fight it. Men are naturally more muscular than women, having approximately ten times as much testosterone. At the risk of seeming redundant, keep those walking shoes laced.

• *Weight gain.* Likely to be temporary, but weight in middle years is always hard to lose, so try to fight it. Avoid flab by choosing the right foods: greens and legumes, fruit and cereal, the right oils (olive is a good one), fish, chicken, and lean beef. For the patient undergoing hormone therapies, stay away from fast food, even if you're feeling sorry for yourself. Keep your metabolism revved and you may not gain too much weight. Don't forget that endorphins (another hormone) are released while you exercise, which just may improve your attitude, thus staving off the desire to overeat.

• *Depression.* This should be temporary but is dangerous, so take precautions. During hormone blockade, depression can be clinically significant—and life-threatening. You and your partner might want to seek therapy, either singly or together. Partner depression, by the way, is also worth discussing. A recent study in *Annals of Behavioral Medicine* examining "Quality of Life of Couples Dealing with Cancer" observed that a partner's psychological distress might drag down the well-being of the cancer patient; the physical health of husbands seems to be especially vulnerable to the poor emotional well-being of their wives.

What is happening to your—or your partner's—body is strange, scary, and confusing. Fight depression any way you can, with therapy, meditation, prayer, conversation, exercise, going for a drive, going to movies, whatever works. Don't be afraid to ask for help. Depression's effect on the spouse or partner may be considerable and is, not surprisingly, intimately connected to the patient's state of mind. In a recent study headlined in *Medical News Today* as "Treating Wife's Stress May Be Indirect Care for Men with Prostate Cancer," Youngmee Kim, director of Family Studies at the American Cancer Society's Behavioral Research Center in Atlanta, noted that helping women manage psychological stress might improve the mental and physical health of both partners. "Men tend not to say that psychological stress associated with cancer diagnosis and treatment is a problem, but they tend to somatize those stresses, reporting headaches, backaches. Maybe men are not conditioned or socialized to express those . . . feelings. They tend to . . . let them come out through their body," Dr. Kim observed.

• *Hot flashes.* Temporary, but possibly appearing ten to twelve times a day. Some men don't get them, but the majority do. Just as women experience them while estrogen wanes, so chemically induced andropause may well do the same. Wearing cool cotton clothes in sheddable layers, drinking water, and avoiding caffeine and alcohol may help.

• *Intestinal discomfort or diarrhea.* This is temporary and often accompanies hot flashes. It is more often associated with anti-androgen pills. Medicines are available; ask your doctor.

• *Loss of libido*. Can be either temporary or permanent; some men don't experience significant changes, while others are changed for life. The relationship between libido and testosterone is not well understood, to date. For the patient, understanding that sexuality is not entirely about "performance" may help. Many men seem to believe that the only sex is Sex, involving firm erections and full penetration. As lethargy sets in, along with fear and uncertainty, libido may wane and, without energetic attempts to preserve it, never reappear. There is, to date, scant sexual counseling available for men about to undergo any of the prostate cancer protocols. Does this bespeak our puritan heritage? I believe it does.

• *Erectile dysfunction*. Can be either temporary or permanent. I read on a Web site of one man who underwent hormone blockade and said that if he had to do it all again, he'd practice in advance of treatment making love with a limp penis! This is to say that performance anxiety often encourages E.D., whether you've had treatments for prostate cancer or are merely middle-aged. Testosterone is not essential to erectile function, but the relationship is unclear. Some men maintain their youthful function, though most lose it for a time. Others enter treatments with a waning function.

According to some studies, more than 80 percent of men report loss of erections at one year following hormone ablation therapy. But there are many devices and drugs to try if your problem does not include libido. Viagra and related drugs will locally increase blood to the penis, thus enabling erection; rings and pumps will do the same thing locally. Injections and penile prostheses are also available. Don't let your doctor ignore this topic.

• *Infertility*. This is likely to be permanent, but miracles do happen. I heard anecdotally of two men who fathered children after hormone ablation therapy, but it is highly unlikely, because testosterone is essential to sperm production. Some men may want to donate sperm to a sperm bank in advance of treatment.

• *Osteoporosis*. After hormone therapy some men suffer from this condition, which has been commonly misconstrued as a "woman's problem." The condition entails loss of bone density, which leads to weakened bones and possible bone breakage. The best way to check bone density is to get a baseline dual energy X-ray absorptiometry scan, or DEXA, and then retest at

165

intervals during and after therapy. Meanwhile, changes in lifestyle are in order. Get plenty of exercise (weight bearing, where possible). Avoid or curtail salty foods, caffeine, and alcohol, and don't smoke. Get enough vitamin D (from modest sun exposure or D-rich foods).

• *"Flare" reaction.* Rare. LHRH analogs may initially cause a flare in testosterone production, which, for men with bone metastases, may be painful. In such cases, an anti-androgen is administered before restarting LHRH.

• *Heart and liver health hazards.* Liver toxicity is a possible side effect of some hormone therapies (2.5 percent of men taking flutamide; 1.4 percent taking bicalutamide). Routine monitoring tests (ALT and AST) detect liver toxicity early in treatment. Preliminary screening for cardiovascular disease with an exercise stress test or accompanying artery classification scan is recommended for patients embarking on hormone therapy.

• *General diminished quality of life.* A buzzword now, "quality of life" was seldom mentioned five years ago. In March 2008, Dr. Martin Sanda, quoting from his recently published article in the *New England Journal of Medicine,* told the *Wall Street Journal:* "Doctors or their patients should think twice if they're considering hormone therapy . . . . Most of the cancers that are treated nowadays are not really that aggressive." What did Dr. Sanda find? "Although each of the three primary therapies for prostate cancer—radiation therapy, brachytherapy, or prostatectomy—appear to be associated with a unique pattern of changes in quality of life, the use of adjuvant hormone therapy may exacerbate events of radiotherapy and brachytherapy."

Dr. Peter Albert's Top Ten List for Prostate Cancer Patients and Their Partners

1. Know the Gleason grade of your tumor, stage of your disease, volume of your disease (how many biopsies were positive and how many were performed), PSA level at time of diagnosis, and size of your prostate gland prior to seeking a consultation with a physician.

2. Get a second or even a third opinion once you have been diagnosed and a treatment regimen has been recommended.

3. Research and study the current literature on prostate cancer, amassing a knowledge base that will help you determine the correct treatment option for you.

4. Attend a meeting of a local prostate cancer support group sponsored by the American Cancer Society, and see how other patients have fared with their treatment choice.

5. Reevaluate your lifestyle: integrate physical healing with a program of dietary and mental health that will make you feel more healthy during your treatment and afterward.

6. Be sensitive in selecting the physician partner who will be there for your treatment and post-treatment care.

7. Undergo any recommended tests, such as bone scan, CT scan, MRI, or lymph node biopsies, in a timely fashion—don't procrastinate.

8. Once treatment is finished, monitor your PSA level every three months for the first year, every six months for the second year, and yearly thereafter.

9. Inform your male blood relatives—sons, brothers, cousins—of your diagnosis, and encourage them to be screened at an early age.

10. Become an active advocate to help other men (and women) who may be beginning their journey in the treatment of prostate cancer.

APPENDIX D

Prostate Cancer Resources and Support Groups

RESOURCES

The following list of resources will be updated yearly on my Web site (www.prostatewife.com).

Advanced Prostate Cancer
Blog.
http://advancedprostatecancer.net/?cat=14

American Cancer Society
With 24-hour hotline.
1-800-ACS-2345
www.cancer.org

> **Cancer Survivors Network**
> www.acscsn.org
>
> **Man to Man**
> National support group network.
> www.cancer.org/docroot/ESN/_3_1x_Man_to_Man_36.asp?sitearea =SHR
>
> Contact the American Cancer Society for information on the Poughkeepsie chapter, which has an excellent newsletter.

American Urological Association
www.urologyhealth.org

Brotherhood of the Balloon
Information and support concerning proton treatments.
www.protonbob.com/proton-treatment-homepage.asp

Canadian Prostate Cancer Network
P.O. Box 1253, Lakefield, ON K0L 2H0
Toll-free 1-866-810-CPCN (2726)
www.cpcn.org

CancerCare
Serves people with cancer and their loved ones throughout
the 50 states, Puerto Rico, and the U.S. Virgin Islands.
275 Seventh Ave., Floor 22, New York, NY 10001
Phone/fax services: 1-800-813-HOPE (4673)
www.cancercare.org

> **CancerCare Education Department**
> Sponsors interesting and free teleconferences, which you
> can join in the privacy of your home.
> teled@cancercare.org

> **Cancer Care E-News**
> info@cancercare.org

Center for Prostate Disease Research
www.cpdr.org

Chemocare.com
www.chemocare.com

C2P (Coach to Player)
Patients and families can ask doctors questions about prostate cancer.
www.pcref.org/c2p.php

Humor and Healing
Humor for the online prostate cancer community.
www.prostatepointers.org/mailman/listinfo/hah

Malecare
Web site of national nonprofit prostate cancer support group network
(including groups for gay prostate cancer patients).
www.malecare.com

National Cancer Institute
NCI Public Inquiries Office, 6116 Executive Blvd., Room 3036A,
Bethesda, MD 20892-8322
1-800-4-CANCER
www.cancer.gov/cancerinfo/types/prostate

National Physician & Family Referral Project
Information on prostate cancer in African-American men.
http://npfrproject.org/

National Prostate Cancer Coalition
Outreach and prostate cancer awareness Web site, a good source
of practical information.
1154 Fifteenth St., NW, Washington, DC 20005
www.fightprostatecancer.org

New York Times
Particularly "Well," a weekly column by Tara Parker-Pope in the Health
section of the Tuesday Science page, which frequently deals with treatment
and post-treatment difficulties of prostate cancer patients and their
partners or families.
well.blogs.nytimes.com

The "New" Prostate Cancer Infolink Social Network
Full of options and information; a real gathering place for men and partners.
prostatecancerinfolink.ning.com

PAACT
Patient Advocates for Advanced Cancer Treatments, Inc.
www.paactusa.org

Patients Helping Patients
Information and advice from one patient to another.
www.prostate-help.org

PCa Women
A group for the spouses and partners of men with prostate cancer.
health.groups.yahoo.com/group/PCa_Women/join?

Phoenix5

"To Help Men and Their Companions Overcome the Effects of Prostate Cancer." The original Phoenix5 site is no longer in existence; for a fascinating and moving explanation of why, see www.phoenix5journal. blogspot.com. The new Phoenix5 is well worth visiting. www.phoenix5.org

> **Prostate Cancer Stages**
> Walks patients through an explanation of staging systems.
> www.phoenix5.org/staging.html

> **A Primer on Prostate Cancer**
> Mostly explains acronyms.
> www.phoenix5.org/Basics/DPprimer0918.html

Prostate Cancer Acronyms and Abbreviations

www.prostatepointers.org/prostate/ed-pip/acronyms.html

Prostate Cancer Action Network

A forum for discussion.
www.prostatepointers.org/mailman/listinfo/pcan

Prostate Cancer and Gay Men

health.groups.yahoo.com/group/prostatecancerandgaymen

Prostate Cancer Foundation of Australia

P. O. Box 1332, Lane Cove NSW 1595, Australia
Toll-free: 1-800-220-099
www.prostate.org.au

Prostate Help—Ladies Only

www.ladies-prostate-forum.org/ladies

Prostate Cancer Research and Education Foundation

www.pcref.org

Prostate Cancer Research Institute

www.prostate-cancer.org

Prostate Cancer Under 50

A group for men diagnosed with prostate cancer age 50 and under, and their families.

www.health.groups.yahoo.com/group/prostatecancerunder50/join

PSA: Prostate Cancer Support Association (U.K.*)*

Membership Secretary, Prostate Cancer Support Association, BM Box 9434, London WC1N 3XX, England

www.prostatecancersupport.co.uk/groups.htm

***PSA Rising* magazine**

www.psa-rising.com

Radiotherapy Clinics of Georgia

Excellent information.

www.rcog.com

Sexual help for couples after prostate disease

www.renewintimacy.org

Surviving Prostate Cancer Without Surgery

www.survivingprostatecancerwithoutsurgery.org

Tom Feeney's Watchful Waiting page

www.prostatepointers.org/ww

**Us TOO International Prostate Cancer Education
& Support Network**

A national prostate cancer support group network that also maintains a lively presence on the Internet.

5003 Fairview Ave., Downers Grove, IL 60515

Phone: 630-795-1002

Fax: 630-795-1602

Hotline: 800-80-UsToo (800-808-7866)

www.ustoo.org

Us TOO ListServs and forums include:

Physician to Patient
www.prostatepointers.org/mailman/listinfo/p2p

NewDx
Offers information and support to those newly diagnosed with prostate cancer.
www.prostatepointers.org/mailman/listinfo/newdx

The Circle
Support for wives, families, friends, and significant others of men with prostate cancer.
www.prostatepointers.org/mailman/listinfo/circle

SeedPods
Mailing list for those interested in brachytherapy as a treatment for prostate cancer.
www.prostatepointers.org/mailman/listinfo/seedpods

RP
Mailing list dedicated to the needs and concerns of patients or prospective patients of radical prostatectomy.
www.prostatepointers.org/mailman/listinfo/rp

IceBalls
Mailing list offering information and support to those interested in cryosurgery for prostate cancer.
www.prostatepointers.org/mailman/listinfo/iceballs

CHB
Discussion and support for patients interested in any form of hormonal blockade.
www.prostatepointers.org/mailman/listinfo/chb

EBRT
Discussion and support for patients interested in any form of radiation therapy for prostate cancer.
www.prostatepointers.org/mailman/listinfo/ebrt

Resource Kit for Making Prostate Cancer Decisions
www.ustoo.org/newpatientkit

WW

Discussion and support for patients interested in active surveillance as a strategy for the management of prostate cancer.
www.prostatepointers.org/mailman/listinfo/ww

Prostate Cancer and Intimacy

ListServ for frank and open discussion of the sexual issues surrounding prostate cancer.
www.prostatepointers.org/mailman/listinfo/pcai

The PCAI list of ED specialists

www.prostatepointers.org/pcai/ed.html

PCAI Wiki

A collaborative treasure trove of knowledge and help from longtime PCAI subscribers. Subscribe to PCAI, then get the wiki URL from the PCAI welcome message.

Spirit

Mailing list for those who want to share spiritual support as they live with prostate cancer.
www.prostatepointers.org/mailman/listinfo/spirit

Promise

Mailing list for those grieving a loss. Also offers help and support to those with a spouse, partner, or family member in the last stages of life.
www.prostatepointers.org/mailman/listinfo/promise

Prostate Problems Mailing List

An unmoderated forum that discusses problems and treatments related to men's prostate gland.
www.ppml-info.org

You Are Not Alone

For prostate cancer patients in Australia and South Africa.
www.yananow.net

What Every Doctor Who Treats Male Patients Should Know

www.yananow.net/DonnasDoctor.html

SUPPORT GROUPS

For the story of the growth of one support group, see *Support Group: A Layman's Service Manual for Surviving Prostate Cancer,* by Dennis O'Hara (founder of Man to Man's Poughkeepsie chapter) and Jules Schwartz, available on Amazon.com. The book includes a chapter by O'Hara's wife, Jackie, the founder of Side by Side.

Certain sites offer online support communites, and a few are for women only. A particularly strong example of an online community is PCa_Women @yahoogroups.com.

Some physical addresses for these organizations are listed under Resources.

Canadian Prostate Cancer Network
www.cpcn.org

MaleCare
www.malecare.com

Outwithcancer
Program for gay, lesbian, bi, and transgender cancer sufferers.
www.outwithcancer.com

Cancermatch
International online support group.
www.cancermatch.com

Man to Man
For men and their partners, but some chapters include only men in monthly meetings. Man to Man is an affiliate of the American Cancer Society.
www.cancer.org/docroot/SHR/content/SHR_2.1_x_Man_to_Man.asp-22k

Us TOO
International organization with 320 chapters worldwide, open to all men, family, friends, and health professionals interested in prostate cancer/ disease. Has an impressive presence on the Internet.
www.ustoo.org

Prostate Cancer Foundation of Australia
www.prostate.org.au/support-groups.php

You Are Not Alone
Australia, South Africa
www.yananow.net

APPENDIX E

On the Horizon

What's on the horizon for prostate cancer patients and partners?

• The Prostate Cancer Foundation (info@prostatecancerfoundation.org) is an excellent source of information on breaking research news. Go to this site for listings of open clinical trials and additional updates.

• A pair of Canadian researchers (Richard Wassersug and John Robinson, with funding from the Canadian Institutes of Health Research) are in the process of launching a program designed to reduce the psychological distress of androgen deprivation therapy for prostate cancer patients and their partners. A major focus of their study and its forthcoming booklet for couples ("A Guide to ADT," soon to be available in the U.S. and Canada) is to determine whether educational intervention about the side effects of ADT (with strategies for overcoming them) can reduce the distress this treatment causes couples.

I have seen a draft copy of this pamphlet and can only say that had it existed when Dean and I were experiencing the results of hormone ablation, it might have changed our lives radically. Sensitively constructed, with helpful questions and suggestions, the pamphlet, which is being used in conjunction with couples workshops, is a shining example of research put to the purpose of humanizing medicine.

For further information, contact:
Richard Wassersug, Ph.D., Department of Anatomy and Neurobiology,
Sir Charles Tupper Medical Building, 5850 College Street, Dalhousie
University, Halifax, Nova Scotia, B3H1X5, Canada

• Vaccine
Prostate-specific membrane antigen DNA vaccine (ultimately for men with metastatic prostate cancer) is currently being studied at Memorial Sloan-Kettering. Follow their Web site (www.mskcc.org) for updates.

GLOSSARY

Active surveillance Also called "watchful waiting," a viable option for men who have decided to observe or monitor their cancer rather than (for the moment) taking any direct treatment action. A PSA blood test and DRE are usually administered every three or four months. If tests indicate that the cancer is growing, treatment may then be initiated. Active surveillance can be a useful tool for men who have very slow growing or early cancers. It may be the best choice for a compliant patient (one willing to be watchful) who has a T1c nonpalpable tumor, a Gleason grade of 6 or less, and a PSA less than 6. Quality-of-life issues often drive the decisions of patients who opt for active surveillance. During active surveillance, a man would also be wise to consider a healthful diet and lifestyle, paying special attention to intake of alcohol, fats, and sugars.

Adrenal gland Endocrine glands located atop each kidney, responsible for producing epinephrine and norepinephrine (adrenaline). The adrenal cortex produces other hormones, including testosterone. Although the prostate is the main source of testosterone, when ADT or hormone therapy is administered, the adrenal gland must also be treated as an auxiliary source of androgens.

ADT *(androgen deprivation therapy—also known as *androgen ablation, hormone ablation, hormone blockade, pulsed androgen ablation)* A (palliative) prostate cancer treatment that eliminates or blocks androgens to the prostate cancer cells. Prostate cancer grows in response to testosterone, which is produced in the testicles and the adrenal gland. This production can be stopped either by removing the testicles (orchiectomy) or via chemical intervention to halt testosterone production (*see anti-androgens and LHRH agonists*); ADT has recently come under fire for its metabolic effects when administered on a continous schedule. Diabetes and cholesterol levels may be exacerbated with continuous (as opposed to "pulsed") use; and increases in life-threatening cardiac and vascular effects (heart attacks, strokes) have been noted in populations of men receiving continuous ADT. Frequent and often lasting side effects, many of which influence quality of life post-treatment, include: reduction of libido (90% in ADT-treated patients), possible E.D. or loss of muscle mass, possible weakness, osteoporosis, shrunken testicles, depression, loss of self-esteem, loss of alertness, and possible loss of higher cognitive functions such as prioritizing. The severity of side effects increases with the length of hormone therapy, which is why "pulsed" androgen ablation may be worth investigating if ADT is called for. ADT is palliative (not curative) because certain cancer cells grow despite the absence of testosterone, so over time the therapy has a less salutary effect.

Androgen ablation (see *ADT*).

Andropause (controversial; also sometimes called *PADAM or "male menopause"*) If it exists, andropause is characterized by a steep drop in testosterone (most men do see testosterone levels drop as they age). For some, these drops are more precipitous than they are for others. Some doctors recognize andropause in patients with low levels of testosterone and prescribe the hormone via patches or injections. Men who have undergone androgen ablation or ADT as part of a prostate cancer treatment protocol may have already experienced something akin to artificially induced andropause; ironically, for them testosterone therapy (patches or shots) is a dangerous concept, as testosterone elimination is part of their treatment.

Anti-androgens Including flutamide (Eulexin or Euflex), bicalutamide (Casodex), and nilutamide (Nilandron), anti-androgens are used in ADT (androgen ablation therapy, which decreases the body's production of testosterone) as a palliative treatment against prostate cancer. These drugs are usually used in combination with luteinizing hormone releasing hormone (LHRH) agonists (Lupron or Zoladex).

Aphrodisiac (controversial) Aphrodisiacs (difficult to document) are substances that, when ingested, supposedly arouse sexual desire or libido. But what is sauce for the goose may very well not be sauce for the gander! In other words, what arouses one sexual partner may have no effect at all upon the other, and what arouses one man may leave the other unmoved. Horny goat weed, Korean red ginseng, yohimbine, and even marijuana have been tried with success by various men. Yohimbine, the product of the bark of an African tree, seems to offer the most promise to date.

Biopsy The removal of pieces of prostate tissue for microscopic examination by a pathologist. The current standard procedure is needle biopsy, in which several tissue samples or cores are removed from different areas of the prostate gland.

Bladder In both male and female bodies, the bladder is the organ in which urine is stored.

Bone scan A bone scan is a test that identifies areas of increased bone metabolism, as well as abnormal processes involving the bone such as tumor, infection, or fracture.

BPH *(benign prostatic hyperplasia)* A condition that affects the prostate gland. The prostate is situated between the bladder (where urine is stored) and the urethra (the tube through which urine passes). As men age, the prostate slowly enlarges and may press on the urethra, which causes the urine flow to be slower and less forceful. The condition is "benign" because the enlargement isn't caused by cancer; it occurs in periurethral glands as opposed to the peripheral zone, where prostate cancer usually arises.

Brachytherapy Sometimes called "seed implantation," brachytherapy is an ultrasonically guided outpatient surgical procedure in which radioactive titanium-coated "seeds" roughly the size of a grain of rice are carefully placed inside the prostate using small needles. The seeds are positioned in order to attack the cancer in a targeted manner and are permanently implanted, although they lose their radioactivity over time. Seeds typically used for treatment include cesium, iodine-125, and palladium-103. The team for implantation includes a urologist (surgeon), a radiation oncologist, and a dosimetrist.

Cancer The uncontrolled growth of abnormal cells in a body, a cancer growth causes destruction to the organ in which it originates; when it spreads, it can eventually kill the entire organism. The malignant tumor will first grow inside the originating organ (e.g., the prostate), then invade the surrounding tissue, blood vessels, or lymph nodes, spreading finally to surrounding tissue and distant sites.

Casodex The brand name for bicalutamide, an anti-androgen sometimes used as part of hormone ablation therapy or androgen ablation (ADT); similar to Eulexin.

Catheter A tube inserted into a body cavity, duct, or vessel, a catheter facilitates drainage of fluids such as urine.

Caverject The brand name for alprostadil, a prescription drug used to treat erectile dysfunction (E.D.) which, when injected into the penis (by a patient, his partner, or a physician), may help to achieve an erection sufficient for intercourse. The needles are similar to needles used by diabetics, and the process is said to be relatively painless when confidently applied.

Cesium The chemical element with the symbol Cs and atomic number 55, a recent addition to the list of choices of radioactive seeds used in brachytherapy.

Cialis The brand name for tadalafil, Cialis is an orally administered drug for treating erectile dysfunction. Tadalafil/Cialis is one of the three chief E.D. prescription drugs in current use; its competitors are sildenafil (Viagra) and vardenafil (Levitra).

Clinical staging In the diagnosis of prostate cancer, the TNM system is the most widely used staging system in the United States. It describes the extent of the primary tumor (T stage), the absence or presence of spread to nearby lymph nodes (N stage), and the absence or presence of metastasis (M stage). This information is gained via PSA, DRE, transrectal ultrasound, and biopsy. Briefly, all stage T1 diagnoses (T1a, T1b, T1c) are not palpable—that is, cannot be felt by an examining doctor during a DRE. T1a and T1b are always found incidentally, whereas T1c is found as the result of an elevated or accelerating PSA, which explains how common this stage is, given the recent wide prevalence of PSA screening. All T2 diagnoses are palpable, but have not yet escaped the prostate capsule. T3 diagnoses have just escaped the capsule. T4 diagnoses have escaped the capsule and seminal vesicles, but are still localized to the pelvic region. For a description of other stages, consult a physician.

Coagulum A soft, insoluble mass formed when a liquid is coagulated.

Cryosurgery (also known as *cryotherapy, cryoablation,* and *cryosurgical ablation*) A surgical procedure in which the prostate gland is frozen under ultrasound-controlled conditions for the purpose of killing cancer cells. Used for many years in the treatment of skin cancer, this procedure is currently considered an experimental therapy for prostate cancer; there are no long-term results to document the technique's effectiveness.

CT scan An effective diagnostic tool for many purposes, computed tomography (CT) uses X rays to make detailed pictures of structures inside the body.

Detrol The brand name for tolterodine, an anticholinergic drug for the relief of urge incontinence. Trospium (Sanctura) is also an anticholinergic.

Diagnosis In medicine, diagnosis (from the Greek, "to know") is the process of identifying a disease by its signs and symptoms, using deductive (eliminative) reasoning, the classic reasoning of all science. (Such is the reasoning beautifully demonstrated in Sherlock Holmes mystery stories, whose author, Sir Arthur Conan Doyle, was a physician.)

Dosimetrist As relates to brachytherapy, a dosimetrist is a member of the radiation oncology team with the expertise to generate radiation dose distributions and dose calculations in collaboration with a radiation oncologist.

DRE *(digital rectal examination)* A simple way to screen for prostate cancer in the early stages, when treatment is most successful. The DRE is typically done during a standard physical exam. Because the prostate lies in front of the rectum, a urologist can feel it by inserting a gloved, lubricated finger into the rectum.

E.D. *(erectile dysfunction)* The clinical and accurate term for what is still widely described as "impotence," E.D. is the inability to achieve or sustain an erection suitable for sexual intercourse. Causes are myriad and sometimes difficult to determine. All major established prostate cancer treatments carry a risk of at least some E.D. And as men age, the probability of E.D. becomes more likely. Conditions such as diabetes, elevated cholesterol, untreated hypertension, poor blood flow to the penis, smoking, drinking alcohol in excess, stress, depression, and hormone ablation are some possible causes.

Eligard (see *luteinizing hormone releasing agonists;* see also *Lupron*) The brand name for one of the LHRH agonists, used in ADT/hormone ablation therapy. These agonists mimic testosterone, convincing the pituitary gland that sufficient testosterone is being manufactured, thus effectively achieving castration levels (90–95% reduction) of the hormone.

Endorphins Neurotransmitters found in the brain with pain-relieving properties similar to morphine. Endorphins interact with opiate-receptor neurons to reduce the intensity of pain. Source of the well-known "runner's high," endorphins are often released during strenuous and prolonged exercise or during sexual activity.

Epididymis A set of tightly coiled tubes located at the top of the testes, which act as a storing place for sperm as they mature.

Erection sufficient for intercourse This phrase has recently come under fire in the dialogue surrounding quality of life for survivors of prostate cancer, specifically as regards erectile dysfunction. According to some researchers, partial or fleeting erections may still be counted in the "success" column.

Eulexin (see also *Casodex*) Brand name for flutamide, an orally active anti-androgen used in hormone ablation (androgen ablation) therapy.

External beam radiation therapy (EBRT) (see also *IMRT, TomoTherapy*) Uses high-energy rays or particles to kill cancer cells. This procedure may be used as the initial treatment for low-grade cancer that is still confined within the prostate gland or that has spread only to nearby tissue, or if the cancer is not completely removed or comes back (recurs) in the area of the prostate after surgery. If the disease is more advanced, radiation may be used to reduce the size of the tumor and to provide relief from present and possible future symptoms. A recent generation of beam radiation (IMRT, TomoTherapy) is more targeted than earlier versions, with the goal of radiating the cancer while sparing the organs (rectum and bladder) situated near the prostate. Treatments involve scheduled visits to a radiation facility.

Flare reaction A transient surge in a patient's concentration of serum testosterone as a result of the use of LHRH agonists.

Flomax Brand name for tamsulosin hydrochloride, an alpha blocker that, by relaxing the muscles of the urinary tract, facilitates urination. It is used to treat the symptoms of an enlarged prostate (benign prostatic hyperplasia, or BPH) and also for men who have difficulty urinating after prostate cancer radiation treatments or for other reasons.

Gleason grade A grading system developed to study the comparative structure of tumor tissue. The ability of a tumor to mimic normal gland architecture is its *differentiation*, and a tumor whose structure is nearly normal (well differentiated) will probably have a biological behavior closer to normal—that is, not aggressively malignant.

A combined grade from two sections of the prostate is usually taken. The lowest possible score is a 2 (1 + 1), where both patterns have a Gleason grade of 1. The highest possible is 10 (5 + 5), when both sections have the greatest de-differentiation from the normal gland architecture.

Half life The life of a quantity (of, say, iodine-125, used in brachytherapy) whose value (in this case, radioactivity) decreases with time after it has decreased to half its initial value.

Hematuria The presence of blood in the urine.

High-dose radiation *(HDR)* A process of treatment by which high-dose iridium rods are drawn through the prostate. A temporary process, as opposed to brachytherapy seed implantation, in which the seeds are permanent.

HIFU *(high-intensity focused ultrasound)* (controversial) A treatment for prostate cancer that is widely practiced outside the U.S. HIFU is lauded by its proponents for its minimally invasive aspects. The procedure utilizes focused sound waves to rapidly heat and destroy the tissue within the prostate. A transrectal probe delivers ultrasound energy directly to the prostate without apparently causing damage to areas outside the gland. This treatment, not currently available in the U.S. (available in Canada, Mexico, and the Caribbean), has created a "medical tourist" effect in certain Mexican resort towns.

IMRT *(intensity modulated radiation therapy; see external beam radiation)*

Iodine-125 The iodine-based seeds used when brachytherapy was originally developed, and still in use today; iodine-125 has a half-life of 60 days.

Kegel exercises An aid to increased continence (and possibly to erectile function), Kegels consist of contracting and relaxing the "pelvic floor" muscles. Traditionally, these exercises include:

Quick pumps: 15 reps, pausing for 30 seconds, then repeating.
Begin at 15 and work up to 100 reps twice daily.
Hold and release: contract the muscle slowly and hold for 5 seconds, release slowly. Work your way to at least 25 reps two times a day.
Elevator: slowly contract 1/3 of the way, pause, then 2/3 of the way, pause, then all the way; 10 reps two times a day.

Laparoscopic radical prostatectomy This form of radical prostatectomy involves inserting a lighted viewing instrument, a laparoscope, into the pelvic region through a tiny incision. In contrast to a traditional (open) prostatectomy, the scar is smaller; thus the operation is said to be less invasive.

LHRH *(luteinizing hormone releasing agonists)* Brand names include: Lupron, Viadur, Zoladex, and Elegard. Used in ADT/hormone ablation therapy, these agents mimic actual hormones, convincing the pituitary gland that sufficient testosterone is being manufactured, thus shutting down the normal production of that hormone.L

Libido Used originally by Freud to signify sexual desire or drive. Of all the terms in the prostate cancer treatment lexicon, *libido* and *erectile dysfunction* (aka "impotence") are perhaps freighted with the greatest significance and are often poorly understood in their differentiation from each other. It is possible for a man to suffer from total erectile dysfunction and still have a sizable libido. Erectile function minus libido is less likely, as libido drives erectile performance. By artificial means such as penile injections, prostheses, or pumps, however, it is possible for a man to achieve an erection without feeling any sexual desire.

Lupron (see *LHRH*)

Male menopause (see *andropause*)

Margins If the pathologist notices that cancer cells are at the very edge of the prostate, touching the ink that was applied during initial processing of the prostate gland, then that "margin" may be said to be positive. Patients with positive surgical margins are at an increased risk of cancer recurrence. Patients with more than one positive margin are at greater risk.

Metastasis The process by which a cancer spreads from the place it first arose in the body as a primary tumor to distant locations.

Nerve-sparing radical prostatectomy A technique used when performing a radical prostatectomy involving sparing the nerve bundles (one on each side of the prostate gland) that allow a man to get and keep an erection, therefore increasing the chances of normal or near-normal erectile function post-treatment.

Nilandron (see *Casodex*) An anti-androgen.

Orchiectomy Surgical castration; the removal of the testicles, the organ that produces 95% of the body's testosterone. (Note that reconstructive surgery—not dissimilar to breast reconstruction—is possible.)

Osteoporosis A disease in which bones become fragile and more likely to break; in the general population, more common in women. It is, however, one possible aftereffect of hormone ablation treatments in men.

Palladium-103 One of the elements used in brachytherapy implantations; it has a half-life of 17 days.

Palliative Any form of medical care or treatment that concentrates on reducing the severity of disease symptoms, rather than attempting to halt, delay, or reverse progression of the disease itself or to provide a cure.

Pelvioscopic assisted radical prostatectomy In this approach to radical prostatectomy, a camera and puncture holes facilitate the removal of the prostate with an instrument called a minilap incisor.

Penile implants Various types of prostheses, the simplest of which consists of a pair of bendable rods surgically implanted within the erection chambers of the penis. With this type of implant, the penis is always semi-rigid and may be adjusted into the erect position at will. Many men choose a hydraulic, inflatable prosthesis, which allows a more natural erection and is much easier to conceal.

Perineum The area of skin located between the scrotum and the anus.

Persistent urinary dysfunction This unfortunate state, which sometimes follows prostate cancer treatments involving radiation, includes urinary incontinence (ranging from some leakage to complete loss of bladder control) and irritative voiding symptoms (including increased frequency, increased urgency, and pain accompanying urination).

Peyronie's disease A connective tissue disorder involving the growth of fibrous plaques in the soft tissue of the penis. Although 1–4% of the general population may experience this disorder, it is also a possible aftereffect of RP (radical prostatectomy). The condition occurs in the tunica albuginea, a fibrous envelope surrounding the penile corpora cavernosa.

Prostate Described typically as a walnut-shaped gland, the prostate lies at the base of the bladder; anterior to the rectum, it encompasses the urethra—a relationship that can aptly be pictured as an orange penetrated through the middle by a straw. Surrounded by a capsule that is as thin as the skin of an onion, the prostate's function is to make fluid that adds vital nutrients to the ejaculate used by the sperm. Functionally, the prostatic glands are divided into an inner and outer group. The inner glands, or the ones surrounding the urethra (called the peri-urethral glands), become enlarged with aging and may give rise to what is called benign hyperplasia or enlargement of the prostate. The outer part of the gland comprises the structures that are most often involved with malignant formation and cancer. The prostate's sexual role has been a source of misinformation among men in particular with regard to libido and potency. The gland functions only as an accessory sexual gland, making fluid to nourish the sperm.

Prostatectomy *(radical prostatectomy, or RP)* The surgical removal of all or part of the prostate gland: this surgery may take various forms, including retropubic, pelvioscopic, laparoscopic, or robotic. All of the above (except for the traditional retropubic) make it possible to concentrate more fully on sparing the nerve bundles that lie on either side of the prostate gland and are essential for erectile function.

Prostate cancer *(PCa)* The uncontrolled growth of cancer cells in the prostate. The cancer is stimulated to grow by testosterone (the male hormone produced in the testis). Cancer of the prostate can be present years before discovery, taking approximately 1 1/2 to 2 years for tumor cells to double in size. Symptoms occur when the prostate enlarges; difficulty in urination may be the first symptom, one that is much more common in benign enlargement of the prostate (see *BPH*). As cancerous cells grow unchecked, they may invade the blood vessels and spread to the vertebral venous system and the bony skeleton, especially the bones of the lumbosacral spine and pelvis. They may also spread to the lymph nodes, traveling often to the lungs and presenting as tumor nodules on a chest X ray. Fifteen to twenty years ago, prior to the present era of PSA screening, bone pain was a very common presenting symptom of prostate cancer. If a tumor can be treated when it is localized, before it has escaped the prostate and especially before it has spread to bone, the physician has the best chance of curing a patient.

Prostatic fluid A whitish secretion that is one of the constituents of semen.

Proton beam therapy Like external beam radiation, proton therapy works by aiming energetic ionizing particles (in this case, protons accelerated with a particle accelerator) onto the target tumor.

PSA screening *(prostate-specific antigen screening)* PSA is a protein produced by the prostate and released in very small amounts into the bloodstream. As prostate cancer develops, more and more PSA is released, until it reaches a level easily detected by a PSA screening (a blood test). PSA levels under 4 ng/mL are generally considered "normal," while over 10 ng/mL are "high" and between 4 and 10 ng/mL are usually considered "intermediate." PSA can also be elevated as a result of BPH or prostatitis. For this reason, a digital rectal exam is also performed at the time of PSA testing.

PSA velocity The rate of rise in PSA level, as followed in PSA-screening blood tests. Recent studies indicate that velocity is a more powerful indicator of eventual recovery or death from prostate cancer than the PSA level itself. These studies seem to indicate that men with a high PSA velocity should not choose "active surveillance" (watchful waiting), as their cancers are likely to be fast-growing. A rapid rise in PSA (20% or more in one year) is likely to indicate that the cancer should be investigated.

Pulsed androgen ablation (see also *ADT*) Hormone ablation administered in six-month cycles, to reduce the drastic systemic effects of long-term treatment.

Pyridium Brand name for phenazopyridine, an analgesic used to relieve urinary pain or burning and increased urge to urinate, sometimes caused by infection or injury, surgery, catheterization, or other conditions that irritate the urinary tract (bladder and urethra).

Quality-of-life issues A current catchphrase in the prostate cancer dialogue that reflects a shift in emphasis, focusing medical and health care interest on survivorship issues. As a result of PSA screening, prostate cancer is more easily diagnosed than it formerly was (thus widening the treatment population and survivorship possibilities), and as the prostate lies at a delicate crossroads of urinary, sexual, and bowel functions in the male body, "quality of life" has recently come to the fore. Currently, all major treatments involve at least some threat to continence, erectile function, and/or libido and affect both patients and partners' quality of life profoundly.

Radiation oncologist A doctor who specializes in the treatment of cancer patients, using radiation as the main modality of treatment.

Robotic prostatectomy An improvement on laparoscopic prostatectomy, this approach employs "the da Vinci," a three-armed robot connected to a remote surgeon console. The surgeon operates the system while seated at the console. The robot has rotation capabilities that mimic the movements of the human wrist. This type of prostatectomy is minimally invasive and has a short learning curve, permitting a surgeon with basic laparoscopic experience to master the method easily.

Salvage surgery Prostate surgery following recurrence of prostate cancer after a previous treatment (usually radiation) has failed. Note: it is particularly difficult to successfully perform a prostatectomy after radiation treatments (since normal tissue planes may already have been obliterated), something younger men considering radiation may want to ponder.

Scrotum A soft, muscular pouch underneath the penis containing two compartments to hold the testicles.

Semen Besides sperm, semen is composed of fluid from the seminal vesicles, the prostate, and the vas deferens. It contains citric acid, free amino acids, fructose, enzymes, phosphorylcholine, prostaglandin, zinc, and potassium.

Seminal vesicles About 5 centimeters long and located behind the bladder and above the prostate, the seminal vesicles contribute fluid to the ejaculate.

Sling A minimally invasive procedure in which a strip of abdominal or synthetic tissue is placed in the pelvis to compress the urethra and prevent urine leakage from stress incontinence. The male sling is a relatively new procedure for men with incontinence as a result of prostate cancer treatment.

Stress incontinence Incontinence resulting from sudden spasm, such as laughing, coughing, or sneezing, resulting in a rise in bladder pressure greater than urethral resting pressure.

Tantric sex Tantra is an Asian body of beliefs and practices that, through ritual, strives to channel the (divine) energy of the universe in refreshing and liberating ways. In the West, Tantric sex has recently taken on special significance as a force in combating aspects of sexual dysfunction. As one of the creative activities or practices that comprise a study of Tantra, certain ritual sexual exercises may help a couple find new ways of approaching intimacy.

Testosterone replacement A series of treatments that may take the form of injections, a patch, gel, or oral tablets, and that provide what is deemed to be adequate levels of replacement testosterone for a man observed to have low testosterone levels. Note that, although some post-treatment prostate cancer survivors have opted for these treatments, *they are considered by most urologists to be a dangerous route for any man who has had prostate cancer and/or treatment for prostate cancer* (testosterone feeds the growth of cancer cells, so may activate dormant cancer cells).

TomoTherapy® (also known as *helical TomoTherapy*) A form of CT-guided IMRT (intensity modulated radiation therapy) that is said to improve upon the model. The advantage of delivering radiation helically (in a CT-like fashion, from 360 degrees) is in the ability to precisely target a tumor while sparing the normal healthy tissue around it. The radiation source rotates around the patient, and so delivers the radiation with precision using many tiny "beamlets."

Urethra In both male and female, the tube through which urine passes.

Urologist (board-certified) In the United States, a physician who has attained certification by the American Board of Urology. He or she has specialized knowledge and skill with regard to problems of the male and female urinary tract and the male reproductive organs. Although classified as a surgical subspecialty, urology, because of the wide variety of clinical problems its practitioners encounter, requires as well a knowledge of internal medicine, pediatrics, gynecology, and other specialties. Note: a non–board certified urologist has completed specialty training in urology after one to two years of general surgery.

Vacuum erection device A device that generates an erection in a man with erectile dysfunction by creating a vacuum. The subject places a plastic cylinder over his penis, thus creating a vacuum by a manual or battery-driven pump; the process brings blood into the penis. He then places an elastic constriction ring at the base of the penis to prevent the blood from returning, and so can maintain an erection safely for up to thirty minutes.

Vas deferens The tube arising from the epididymis that conducts sperm produced in the testes into the ejaculatory duct.

Viagra Chief brand name for sildenafil citrate, a drug used to treat male erectile dysfunction and pulmonary arterial hypertension. The "little blue pill" acts by inhibiting an enzyme that regulates blood flow to the penis. Similar drugs on the market currently include tadalafil (Cialis) and vardenafil (Levitra). Note: as erectile dysfunction and libido are not synonymous, Viagra and its equivalents may work best where libido has not been affected. Patients with vision problems, such as macular degeneration, or pulmonary complications may be at risk taking these medicines.

Watchful waiting (see *active surveillance*)

Yohimbine (see also *aphrodisiac*) Derived from the bark of an African tree, yohimbine has been said to be a true aphrodisiac. Regardless of whether it lives up to this reputation, doctors have used it for many years to treat certain cases of E.D. It is thought that yohimbine works by increasing sensation to areas of the brain that govern libido.

Zoladex (see *LHRH*)

BIBLIOGRAPHY

Auden, W. H. "Musée des Beaux Arts." In *Selected Poems, New Edition*. New York: Vintage Books/Random House, 1979.

Berberich, Ralph. *Hit Below the Belt*. Berkeley, CA: Celestial Arts, 2001.

Blum, Deborah. *Sex on the Brain: The Biological Differences Between Men and Women*. New York: Penguin Putnam, 1997.

Bordo, Susan. *The Male Body: A New Look at Men in Public and in Private*. New York: Farrar, Straus, and Giroux, 1999.

Brown, Lesley, ed. *The New Shorter Oxford English Dictionary*. Oxford, U.K.: Oxford University Press, 2002.

DeBeauvoir, Simone. *The Second Sex*. New York: Vintage Books, 1989.

Donne, John. "A Valediction: Forbidding Mourning." In *John Donne's Poetry*, ed. A. L. Clements. New York: Norton, 1966.

Gordon, Judy, and Dan Gordon. *The Heroics of Falling Apart: One Couple's Breast Cancer Journey*. iUniverse, 2007.

Groopman, Jerome. *How Doctors Think*. Boston: Houghton Mifflin, 2007.

———. *Second Opinions*. New York: Viking, 2000.

Hite, Shere. *The Hite Report on Male Sexuality*. New York: Knopf, 1981.

Justman, Stewart. *Seeds of Mortality: The Public and Private Worlds of Cancer*. Chicago: Ivan R. Dee, 2003.

Kinsey, Alfred Charles, Wardell B. Pomeroy, and Clyde E. Martin, *Sexual Behavior in the Human Male*. Reprinted. Bloomington: Indiana University Press, 1998.

Korda, Michael. *Man to Man*. New York: Random House, 1996.

Michael, Robert T., John H. Gagnon, Edward O. Lauman, and Gina Kolata. *Sex in America*. New York: Warner Books, 1994.

O'Hara, Dennis, and Jules Schwartz. *Support Group*. SJDJ Inc., 1997.

Propp, Karen. *In Sickness and in Health*. Rodale Press, 2002.

Remen, Rachel Naomi, M.D. *Kitchen Table Wisdom: Stories That Heal*. New York: Riverhead Books, 2006.

Roth, Philip. *Exit Ghost*. New York: Houghton Mifflin, 2007.

Rosenblatt, Paul C. *Two in a Bed: The Social System of Couple Bed Sharing.* Albany: State University of New York Press, 2006.

Sontag, Susan. *AIDS and Its Metaphors.* New York: Picador, 2001.

———. *Illness as Metaphor.* New York: Picador, 2001.

Tiefer, Leonore. *Sex Is Not a Natural Act.* Boulder, CO: Westview Press, 2004.

Wainrib, Barbara Rubin, and Sandra Haber. *Men, Women, and Prostate Cancer: A Medical and Psychological Guide for Women and the Men They Love.* Oakland, CA: New Harbinger Publications, 2000.

Walsh, Patrick. *The Prostate: A Guide for Men and the Women Who Love Them.* Baltimore: Johns Hopkins University Press, 1995.

ACKNOWLEDGMENTS

For my husband, Dean, who stuck with this project.

If it hadn't been for a certain group—half of them poets, half prose writers—this book probably wouldn't have grown from my journals and essays into its current form. One woman in particular, Nancy Kline, a brilliant fiction writer (who has served as a prose mentor to me), deserves particular thanks for responding with enthusiasm to journal excerpts I presented in that group. Thanks also to the other members of this group: Susan Sindall, as excellent a friend as she is a poet, and Polly Howells, a new friend and a prose writer of talent and depth.

Thanks to Peggy Anderson, good friend and mentor, a prose writer whose work I greatly admire, and to Fredi Friedman, my agent, for being so stubborn and smart, for seeing this book and helping it to find its home. That home, at Newmarket Press, has turned out to be an excellent one, indeed: thanks so much to my publisher, Esther Margolis, for her wisdom, for seeing immediately the worth of this project, and to my excellent and tactful editor, Linda Carbone, for helping me bring the book to completion. Thanks also to Keith Hollaman, Heidi Sachner, and Harry Burton.

Without the expert guidance and friendship of Dr. Peter Albert, the urologist we wish we'd known sooner, and his wife, Elaine Albert, a nurse and talented support group facilitator, this book would have been limited, indeed. As health care professionals who also happen to be a cancer survivor (Elaine) and the partner of a cancer survivor (Peter), they are uniquely suited to understand this book's mission and perspective.

Thanks to the American Cancer Society, where our group,

What About Me?, found a home.

To the wives and partners of prostate cancer survivors who agreed to be interviewed for this book, thanks for your courage. Their names have been changed, which enabled them to speak freely. There are women I will never meet whose postings on certain sites helped frame the way I think about particular issues, and whose honesty and commitment to the prostate cancer community have helped me feel that we are not alone.

To my sister Judy Borie for exclaiming, after finding an early manuscript, "This is the story of a marriage!"

To my friends who have been readers and advisers: Michael Carman and Peggy Garrison, thank you for wanting to read and for your enthusiasm. Thanks also to Michael for her professional proofreading skills. My workshop group from the summer of 2007, "Writing the Medical Experience," at Sarah Lawrence College, was wonderfully supportive: thanks for saying that chapter 1 stands by itself, and for wanting to meet Dean after reading his voice! Thanks to David Watts for his wise counsel during the conference.

Thanks to Denise Sender-Vinograde for insisting that this book will have a life of its own.

I owe a special thanks to members of our Staten Island partners-of-cancer-survivors group, *What About Me?*, whose stories keep reminding me how different every individual and every cancer is, and how elaborate the network of family and friends can be.

To Man to Man (both our local group in Staten Island and the Poughkeepsie chapter—Dennis and Jackie and everyone there), thanks for welcoming me and for showing me the strength of community.

Finally, thanks to my poetry group: Priscilla Ellsworth, Sabra Loomis, Myra Shapiro, Mary Jane Nealon, and Wendy Wilder Larson, for all your encouragement, and to Sabra especially for giving me the sentence that started this book: "They can save us, if we're lucky, but then how do we deal with surviving the cure?"

INDEX

D

de Beauvoir, Simone, 106
depression, 27, 73, 106, 164
Detrol, 114
diagnosis, 10–14, 15–16
  via biopsy, 11, 12
  first month after, 24–36
diarrhea, 164
doctors. *See* physicians
domestic effects of cancer. *See* life of
  couple
Donne, John, 81
dosimetrist, 86

E

emotions
  anger, 12–13, 75, 100–102
  bargaining, 75
  couple's life together (*See* life of
    couple)
  denial, 75
  false bravado, 38, 39–40
  mood swings and depression, 3,
    27, 73–74, 77–79, 106, 164
  preparation for changes, 64
  self-pity, 38–39
  spouse's search for community,
    55–56, 57
  support group (*See* support net-
    work)
erectile function, 28, 40, 49, 50, 65
  age at loss, 71
  brachytherapy, effects of, 122–23,
    157
  confusion in results, 122–23
  external beam radiation, effect of,
    156

getting back, 132–38
HIFU and, 158
hormone ablation effect on, 4,
  158, 165
impotence question, 129–31
incontinence, tradeoff with,
  130–31
prostatectomy, after, 63, 155
questioning doctor about, 64
scarring, effects of, 1, 2, 87
suggestions for increasing,
  136–37
exercise, importance of, 104–5
Exit Ghost (Roth), 71, 126
external beam radiation, 2–3, 18,
  30, 66–67, 156. *See also* IMRT
  and erectile dysfunction, chances
    of, 156
  hypothetical case history of, 70
  and incontinence, chances of,
    127, 155
  side effects of, 156
  technique of, 156

F

false bravado, 38, 39–40
Faulkner, William, 110
"flare" reaction, 166
Flomax, 114, 126, 128

G

Giuliani, Rudy, 26
Glacier National Park, 10–11
Gleason grades, 29, 30, 38, 65, 167
  meaning of, 159
Gordon, Judy, 115

ABOUT THE AUTHOR

VICTORIA HALLERMAN is a published poet and educational literacy consultant with an abiding interest in health issues. She and Dean have been married since 1969. His prostate cancer diagnosis and treatment, difficult as they may have been, changed the landscape of their life together and altered the course of her own career. Now to her credentials as educator and poet, she adds health activist.

Through her involvement in the cancer community, she has become a member of Man to Man, the national prostate cancer support group network. This involvement led her to co-found a support group of wives and partners of prostate cancer survivors. With her local chapter of the American Cancer Society, she and a colleague have recently founded What About Me?, a group for partners of patients with all forms of cancer who have become survivors.

Victoria has been a poet for over twenty years. Her previous book, *The Aerialist* (Bright Hill Press, 2005), was the winner of the Bright Hill Prize. Her work has appeared in numerous literary journals and magazines, including *Poetry* (where she has been a regular contributor since 1984), *The Nation, The Indiana Review, Global City Review, The Los Angeles Review,* and *Runes.* In 1990, she won Discovery/*The Nation,* given by *The Nation* and the 92nd Street Y in New York City. Her work has been anthologized in *The Pushcart Prize: Best of the Small Presses,* and is included in the permanent archive of the Academy of American Poets.

For more information on Victoria's work, both as a health advocate and as a poet, visit www.victoriahallerman.com.

PETER S. ALBERT, M.D., F.A.C.S., has been attending urologist/surgeon at Staten Island University Hospital since 1975 and is also in private practice. He is the author of more than 30 articles in medical journals and has contributed chapters to several books on endoscopic and laparoscopic surgery.

Health Books
from Newmarket Press

Available wherever books are sold or directly from the publisher.

Outliving Heart Disease: The 10 New Rules for Prevention and Treatment, *by Richard A. Stein, M.D.*

__Copies at $16.95 (paperback) 978-1-55704-788-5
__Copies at $24.95 (hardcover) 978-1-55704-594-2

How We Survived Prostate Cancer: What We Did and What We Should Have Done, *by Victoria Hallerman, Foreword by Peter S. Albert, M.D.*

__ Copies at $16.95 each (paperback) 978-1-55704-819-6
__ Copies at $24.95 each (hardcover) 978-1-55704-814-1

When Someone You Love Needs Nursing Home, Assisted Living, or In-Home Care, Revised Second Edition, *by Robert Bornstein, Ph.D., and Mary A. Languirand, Ph.D.*

__ Copies at $16.95 each (paperback) 978-1-55704-816-5
__ Copies at $24.95 each (hardcover) 978-1-55704-822-6

The Antioxidant Save-Your-Life Cookbook: 150 Nutritious, High-Fiber, Low-Fat Recipes to Protect You Against the Damaging Effects of Free Radicals, *by Jane Kinderlehrer and Daniel A. Kinderlehrer, M.D.*

__ Copies at $16.95 (paperback) 978-1-55704-760-1

The Dorm Room Diet: The 8-Step Program for Creating a Healthy Lifestyle Plan That Really Works, *by Daphne Oz, Foreword by Mehmet Oz, M.D.*

__ Copies at $16.95 each (paperback) 978-1-55704-685-7

The Dorm Room Diet Planner, *by Daphne Oz*

__ Copies at $12.95 (paperback) 978-1-55704-761-8

Discovering the Power of Self-Hypnosis: The Simple, Natural Mind-Body Approach to Change and Healing, Second Expanded Edition, *by Stanley Fisher, Ph.D., Foreword by Gail Sheehy*

__ Copies at $14.95 each (paperback) 978-1-55704-502-7
__ Copies at $24.95 each (hardcover) 978-1-55704-361-0